COVID-19 and Pandemic Preparedness: Lessons Learned and Next Steps

Editor

KELLY A. WOLGAST

NURSING CLINICS
OF NORTH AMERICA

www.nursing.theclinics.com

Consulting Editor
BENJAMIN SMALLHEER

March 2023 • Volume 58 • Number 1

ELSEVIER

1600 John F. Kennedy Boulevard • Suite 1800 • Philadelphia, Pennsylvania, 19103-2899

http://www.theclinics.com

NURSING CLINICS OF NORTH AMERICA Volume 58, Number 1
March 2023 ISSN 0029-6465, ISBN-13: 978-0-323-93973-7

Editor: Kerry Holland
Developmental Editor: Axell Ivan Jade M. Purificacion

Nursing Clinics of North America (ISSN 0029-6465) is published quarterly by Elsevier Inc., 360 Park Avenue South, New York, NY 10010-1710. Months of issue are March, June, September, and December. Periodicals postage paid at New York, NY and additional mailing offices. Subscription price per year is, $163.00 (US individuals), $557.00 (US institutions), $275.00 (international individuals), $680.00 (international institutions), $231.00 (Canadian individuals), $680.00 (Canadian institutions), $100.00 (US and Canadian students), and $135.00 (international students). To receive student/resident rate, orders must be accompanied by name of affiliated institution, date of term, and the signature of program/residency coordinator on institution letterhead. Orders will be billed at individual rate until proof of status is received. Foreign air speed delivery is included in all *Clinics* subscription prices. All prices are subject to change without notice. **POSTMASTER:** Send address changes to *Nursing Clinics*, Elsevier Health Sciences Division, Subscription Customer Service, 3251 Riverport Lane, Maryland Heights, MO 63043. **Customer Service: Telephone: 1-800-654-2452** (U.S. and Canada); **1-314-447-8871 (outside U.S. and Canada). Fax: 1-314-447-8029. E-mail: journalscustomerservice-usa@ elsevier.com** (for print support) and **journalsonlinesupport-usa@elsevier.com** (for online support).

Nursing Clinics of North America is covered in *EMBASE/Excerpta Medica, MEDLINE/PubMed (Index Medicus), Social Sciences Citation Index, Current Contents, ASCA, Cumulative Index to Nursing, RNdex Top 100,* and Allied Health Literature and International Nursing Index (INI).

Contributors

CONSULTING EDITOR

BENJAMIN SMALLHEER, PhD, RN, ACNP-BC, FNP-BC, CCRN, CNE
Associate Clinical Professor, School of Nursing, Duke University, Durham, North Carolina, USA

EDITOR

KELLY A. WOLGAST, DNP, RN, FACHE, FAAN
COL (R), US Army, Associate Teaching Professor and Assistant Dean for Outreach and Professional Development, Ross and Carol Nese College of Nursing, Director, Penn State COVID-19 Operations Control Center, The Pennsylvania State University, University Park, Pennsylvania, USA

AUTHORS

SAMANTHA ACRI, MPH
Systems Analyst Intermediate, Center for Quality Innovation, Penn State Health Shared Services, Hershey, Pennsylvania, USA

RACHEL ALLEN, PhD, PMHNP-BC, RN
Assistant Research Professor, College of Nursing, The Pennsylvania State University, Hershey, Pennsylvania, USA

SARA BANO, PhD
Assistant Professor, School of Education, North Dakota State University, Fargo, North Dakota, USA

JENNIFER BARTON, DNP, RN, CNE, WHNP-BC
Assistant Teaching Professor, Nursing Program Coordinator, The Pennsylvania State University, Ross and Carol Nese College of Nursing, Hershey Campus, Hershey, Pennsylvania, USA

MARIE BOLTZ, PhD, GNP-BC, FGSA, FAAN
Elouise Ross Eberly and Robert Eberly Professor, Ross and Carol Nese College of Nursing, Penn State, University Park, Pennsylvania, USA

PETRA BRYSIEWICZ, PhD
Professor, School of Nursing and Public Health, University of KwaZulu-Natal, Glenwood, Durban, South Africa

JENNIFER CHIPPS, PhD
Professor, School of Nursing, Faculty of Community and Health Sciences, University of the Western Cape, Belville, Cape Town, South Africa

COLLETTE CHRISTOFFERS, MSN, RN, PHN, CNE
EdD Graduate Student, School of Education, North Dakota State University, Fargo, North Dakota, USA

ZAHARAA DAVOOD, MPH
Pennsylvania Action Coalition Senior Manager, National Nurse-Led Care Consortium - Pennsylvania Action Coalition, Philadelphia, Pennsylvania, USA

MICHAEL M. EVANS, PhD, MSEd, RN, ACNS, CMSRN, CNE
Assistant Dean of Undergraduate Nursing Education at the Commonwealth Campuses, Teaching Professor of Nursing, The Pennsylvania State University, Ross and Carol Nese College of Nursing, Dunmore, Pennsylvania, USA

LORI A. FRANCIS, PhD
Associate Professor, Department of Biobehavioral Health, The Pennsylvania State University, University Park, Pennsylvania, USA

CHRISTOPHER M. GARRISON, PhD, RN, CNE, CHSE
The Ross and Carol Nese College of Nursing, The Pennsylvania State University, University Park, Pennsylvania, USA

JENNIFER GIMBEL, MBA
Pennsylvania Action Coalition Director, National Nurse-Led Care Consortium - Pennsylvania Action Coalition, Philadelphia, Pennsylvania, USA

KRISTINE GONNELLA, MPH
Strategy Development, Public Health Management Corporation, College of Public Health, Temple University, Philadelphia, Pennsylvania, USA

MELISSA GORZ, MEd
PhD Graduate Student, School of Education, North Dakota State University, Fargo, North Dakota, USA

MONICA HARMON, MSN, MPH, RN
Drexel University, College of Nursing and Health Professions Community Wellness HUB, Pennsylvania Action Coalition, Nurse Diversity Council, Dornsife Center for Neighborhood Partnerships, Philadelphia, Pennsylvania, USA

KRISTAL HOCKENBERRY, MSN, RN, CNE, CDP
The Ross and Carol Nese College of Nursing, The Pennsylvania State University, University Park, Pennsylvania, USA

SARAH HEXEM HUBBARD, JD
Executive Director, National Nurse-Led Care Consortium, Philadelphia, Pennsylvania, USA

CATHERINE H. IVORY, PhD, RN-BC, NEA-BC, FAAN
Associate Nurse Executive, Practice Excellence, Vanderbilt University Medical Center, Nashville, Tennessee, USA

MARY LOUISE KANASKIE, PhD, RN, NPD-BC
Director, Office of Nursing Research and Innovation, Penn State Health Milton S. Hershey Medical Center, Hershey, Pennsylvania, USA

KALEI KOWALCHIK, BSN, RN
BSN-PhD Student, Graduate Fellow, The Pennsylvania State University, Ross and Carol Nese College of Nursing, University Park Campus, Olyphant, Pennsylvania, USA

SHARON LACUE, DNP, RN, CNE, CHSE
The Ross and Carol Nese College of Nursing, The Pennsylvania State University,
University Park, Pennsylvania, USA

DEEPA MANKIKAR, MPH
National Nurse-Led Care Consortium, Philadelphia, Pennsylvania, USA

KRISTI MATTZELA, MSW, LSW
Clinical Services Director, Centre Volunteers in Medicine, State College, Pennsylvania,
USA

KIERNAN RILEY, PhD, RN
Assistant Professor, Fitchburg State University, Worcester, Massachusetts, USA

CYNTHIA K. SNYDER, PhD, RN
Assistant Professor of Nursing, Eastern University, St Davids, Elizabethtown,
Pennsylvania, USA

CATHERINE STILLER, PhD, RN, CNE
Assistant Teaching Professor, The Pennsylvania State University, Ross and Carol Nese
College of Nursing, Erie, The Behrend College, Erie, Pennsylvania, USA

KIMBERLY STREIFF, DEd, MSN, CCRN, CRNP, FNP-C, CNE
Assistant Teaching Professor, Nursing Program Coordinator, The Pennsylvania State
University, Ross and Carol Nese College of Nursing, Erie, The Behrend College, Edinboro,
Pennsylvania, USA

PHILIP D. WALKER, MLIS, MS
Director, Annette and Irwin Eskind Family Biomedical Library and Learning Center,
Vanderbilt University, Nashville, Tennessee, USA

CHERYL JO WHITE, RN
Executive Director, Centre Volunteers in Medicine, State College, Pennsylvania, USA

Contents

> Nursing education faced unprecedented challenges in maintaining quality clinical and simulation instruction during the COVID-19 pandemic. Strategies to maintain clinical engagement and meet course objectives included using virtual simulation and safely reopening simulation laboratories as soon as it was possible. When using virtual experiences for replacement of clinical or simulation, it is critical that standards of best practice are implemented. Safely reopening laboratories required plans for social distancing, health screening, personal protective equipment, disinfecting, and educating users on the new protocols. Combining these strategies resulted in delivering quality instruction without interruption during the pandemic.

> A free and charitable clinic successfully designed and implemented mass COVID-19 vaccination clinics in a semirural area in Central Pennsylvania. A total of 172 clinics were offered, approximately 500 volunteers were mobilized, and approximately 45,000 vaccine doses were administered. Partnering with local schools, universities, and recreation centers to offer mass vaccination clinics made it possible to expand the clinic's reach beyond its own patients. Findings provide evidence for the capacity of small community clinics to respond to major public health emergencies, such as a pandemic.

> The coronavirus disease-2019 pandemic disrupted traditional research practices with the cessation of face-to-face contact with study participants. Researchers needed to respond with alternative methods to continue nurse-led clinical research. A rapid pivot to remote processes for recruitment, enrollment, data collection, and participant incentives can enable research to continue despite restrictions on in-person activities. Technology offers innovative methods in meeting current research needs but is not without challenges and continued need for ethics evaluation.

> US nursing homes and other long-term care (LTC) communities such as assisted living and adult day care services have been disproportionally affected by COVID-19. Nurses and health care workers provided care and services despite health concerns for themselves and family members. Nurses on the frontline were called to act with extraordinary tenacity, skill, flexibility, and creativity to prevent infection; prevent complications; and optimize function, health, and well-being. The purpose of this article is to provide an overview of the challenges posed by the COVID-19 pandemic and the strategies prioritized and implemented by nurse and interdisciplinary colleagues in LTC settings.

> At the height of the COVID-19 pandemic, faculty, staff, and administrators at a large research university in the mid-Atlantic part of the country pivoted to move many classes, laboratories, and clinical experiences to a virtual environment to mitigate the risks of COVID-19. This article will highlight 2 exemplars of how faculty at this university provided students with options to learn in-person or online and how faculty managed to provide students with valuable online learning experiences. Through innovative teaching strategies, this university was able to graduate competent nurses when they were most needed by society.

 Video content accompanies this article at http://www.nursing.theclinics.com.

> This article describes how coronavirus disease 2019 (COVID-19) health disparities relate to the social determinants of health and reviews the importance of a diverse nursing workforce prepared to advance social justice. The article reviews recommendations from the National Academy of Medicine and highlights practical strategies to promote diversity and social justice, including mentoring nurses from underrepresented backgrounds, amplifying diverse nursing voices, and leveraging the power of coalitions. In highlighting the interwoven impact of COVID-19 and demand for social change throughout 2020 to 2022, the article strives to move beyond the acute COVID-19 crisis to sustained social justice in health care.

> Nurses are recognized as trusted messengers, yet there is an absence of nurse presence in media. The coronavirus disease 2019 (COVID-19) pandemic provided an opportunity to encourage vaccine confidence and increase COVID-19 vaccines through leveraging the trusted voice of

nurses through social media. The COVID-19 vaccine confidence social media campaign highlighted an emerging opportunity for nurses to create and promote public policy, have more visibility in media, and maximize their role as trusted messengers in health care.

NURSING CLINICS

SERIES OF RELATED INTEREST

Advances in Family Practice Nursing
www.advancesinfamilypracticenursing.com

THE CLINICS ARE AVAILABLE ONLINE!
Access your subscription at:
www.theclinics.com

Foreword

Learning from the Past to Grow the Future

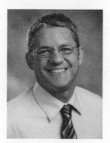

Benjamin Smallheer, PhD, RN, ACNP-BC, FNP-BC, CCRN, CNE
Editor

March of 2020 brought about health care concerns that most Baby Boomers and Generations X, Y, and Z never could have imagined needing to endure. The COVID-19 pandemic forced an evaluation of personal relationships, work structures, and life boundaries. As more time passes between present day and this global event of 2020 to 2021, memories of the challenges and struggles the profession of nursing encountered will likely mature.

New York Times author, Lauren Hilgers,[1] wrote a stunning piece titled, "Nurses have finally learned what they're worth" (February 15, 2022), which captures the essence of culture shifts within nursing because of extreme distress both within the work environment and at home. Ms Hilgers illuminates the life events of several bedside nurses and their struggles during times of low staffing, ethical dilemma, and emotional burnout, which have all led to changes in the way nurses viewed their work and, essentially, their worth.

Within nursing education, faculty who were engaged in any aspect of face-to-face instruction scrambled to move all content into a fully online format with a strong degree of virtual presence without lessening the quality of nursing education. In addition, most precepted learning experiences and clinical placements were abruptly halted for nursing students. These challenges catalyzed a high degree of innovation from the world of nursing academia to assure students within schools of nursing worldwide did not experience a halt in their academic progression.

Meanwhile, back at the point of impact, communities and the health care system were rocked with unprecedented instability. Leadership was challenged; the trajectory of patient care was unsure, and mechanisms of care delivery to all age ranges were actively being reimaged. As a global community of nurses, we would have never imagined the unsteady footing we were experiencing.

Nurs Clin N Am 58 (2023) xi–xii
https://doi.org/10.1016/j.cnur.2022.12.001
0029-6465/23/© 2022 Published by Elsevier Inc.

So, what have we learned? At the time this issue is published, we are nearly one year out from the pandemic being declared over by global experts. Thus, these articles serve as a time capsule capturing our immediate reflections of the two-year period that significantly changed the nursing profession. We learned how to be stronger, teach differently, and grow more efficiently, and more importantly, we have learned our worth. Guest edited by my friend and colleague, Dr Kelly Wolgast, this issue of *Nursing Clinics of North America* provides a snapshot into our immediate reflection. The lessons learned, though not all inclusive, will help guide us toward emergency preparedness for the next global pandemic; we know it will happen one day. It is inevitable. Our lessons learned and next steps will assure we continue to grow as a profession and as a global community.

Benjamin Smallheer, PhD, RN, ACNP-BC, FNP-BC, CCRN, CNE
School of Nursing
Duke University
307 Trent Drive
DUMC Box 3322, Office 3117
Durham, NC 27710, USA

E-mail address:
benjamin.smallheer@duke.edu

REFERENCE

1. Hilgers L. Nurses have finally learned what they're worth. New York Times 2022. Available at: https://www.nytimes.com/2022/02/15/magazine/traveling-nurses.html. Accessed December 10, 2022.

Preface

Resilient Nurses Doing What Is Necessary to Protect Patients and Communities During COVID-19

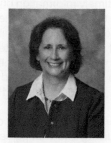

Kelly A. Wolgast, DNP, RN, FACHE, FAAN
Editor

Nurses around the world absorbed the numerous impacts of the SARS-CoV-2 (COVID-19) pandemic in all settings in which nurses lead and deliver care. In this issue of *Nursing Clinics of North America*, the focus is to highlight innovation, resilience, grit, perseverance, and lessons learned that emerged out of necessity as nurses quickly learned how to adapt to this dangerous novel virus. Nurses in current practice in various care settings and environments along with nurse educators and nursing students in all levels of educational programs were forced to navigate rapid changes in care requirements not experienced before in such magnitude.

Disruptions during COVID-19 affected clinical environments, community care and outreach, social justice efforts, long-term care, traditional nursing education methods, and nursing research efforts, and strained long-standing nursing processes related to supporting and maintaining a healthy nursing workforce. The articles in this issue cover a spectrum of lessons learned to codify that learning for when we encounter the next global health emergency. Two of the articles presented by nurse educators share how they adapted learning environments for nursing faculty and students to maintain high-quality education activities while incorporating COVID-19 mitigations, such as physical distancing, masking, and rigorous disinfecting, in simulation centers of learning and in modified or restricted clinical experiences. Nurse educators also quickly adapted learning methodologies to online forums to minimize any delays in student progression. Nurse researcher colleagues share how they adopted alternative methods to continue important recruitment, enrollment, data collection, and timeline management for ongoing research efforts. Nurses providing care to vulnerable patients in long-term care, the population that bore disproportionate impact by the pandemic, discuss strategies to optimize function, health, and well-being through demonstrated extraordinary

Nurs Clin N Am 58 (2023) xiii–xiv
https://doi.org/10.1016/j.cnur.2022.11.002
0029-6465/23/© 2022 Published by Elsevier Inc.

resilience. Health care leaders from the Pennsylvania Action Coalition present thoughts on practical strategies to promote diversity and social justice within nursing and health care, highlighting the impact from COVID-19, and importantly, the need for sustained focus on diversity, inclusion, and belonging in the nursing workforce. Colleagues in a free and charitable clinic present a success story in the volume of COVID-19 vaccination clinics that they were able to plan and execute with help from partnering local champions—demonstrating that with vision and leadership, population health response can be expansive. Technology innovations served to assist the nursing workforce during the pandemic. One article covers the development of a web-based solution to help nurses better locate and organize timely information on how to best care for patients and themselves. Nurses' visibility in the media also gained spotlight attention at the national level in the United States. One article shares details about a social media campaign developed to raise the voices of nurses and promote nurses as reliable sources of information. Emphasizing the global reach of nursing, colleagues from South Africa contribute perspective on how best to document the lived experiences of nurses to call attention to the contributions and value of nurses and nursing to the world.

All the authors who contributed to this issue experienced the pandemic in a different way and led efforts to ensure that the work they do in Nursing and with nurses made responsive changes as swiftly as possible to meet the dynamic conditions forced by the pandemic. Nurses around the world learned to apply every skill possible to determine and enact the very best solutions. I, for one, changed roles when selected to lead and direct the COVID-19 operations at The Pennsylvania State University, a land-grant, public research university with nearly 100,000 students from over 130 countries globally and 37,000 employees across 24 campuses. That work has continued for over 2½ years with an amazing team of Penn State professionals assisting me. As I was grounded by my experience in the US Army and by my foundational leadership experiences in nursing, health care, and academia, dedicating that level of effort in service as a nurse leader to my university community was and continues to be a great honor. I hope that this issue will inspire other nurses to write about their experiences from the pandemic so that we capture more of the lessons learned to share with those who follow in our nursing footsteps. Our lives and those of our patients, families, friends, neighbors, and communities are forever changed.

Kelly A. Wolgast, DNP, RN, FACHE, FAAN
COL (R), US Army
Ross and Carol Nese College of Nursing
Penn State COVID-19 Operations Control Center
The Pennsylvania State University
University Park, PA 16802, USA

E-mail address:
kaw466@psu.edu

Adapting Simulation Education During a Pandemic

Christopher M. Garrison, PhD, RN, CNE, CHSE*,
Kristal Hockenberry, MSN, RN, CNE, CDP,
Sharon Lacue, DNP, RN, CNE, CHSE

KEYWORDS

- Simulation during COVID • Nursing education • Virtual simulation
- Simulation infection control

KEY POINTS

- Rapidly transitioning nursing education during the COVID-19 required the strategic use of virtual simulation and plans to safely return to face-to-face instruction in the simulation laboratory.
- When changing instructional delivery, such as going from in-person clinical or high-fidelity simulation to virtual simulation, standards of best practice need to be followed.
- Infection control considerations for simulation during the pandemic include social distancing, screening for laboratory entry, personal protective equipment, disinfecting surfaces and equipment, and informing stakeholders about the guidelines.
- When making rapid changes in instructional strategies, as was required during the pandemic, it is critical to have a plan to evaluate instruction to ensure that learning objectives are being met.

INTRODUCTION

In March 2020, the World Health Organization (WHO) declared novel coronavirus (COVID-19) to be a global pandemic.[1] Nursing education was faced with unprecedented challenges in response to the pandemic. Nursing programs discontinued in-person instruction and clinical sites closed to students.[2,3] In response, learning had to be transitioned online. Delivering nursing curricula online is particularly challenging due to the need for students to interact with patients and practice psychomotor skills.[4] Virtual simulation was used broadly throughout the country to replace in-person simulation and clinical.[2,5] A national survey of pre-licensure nursing students who

The Ross and Carol Nese College of Nursing, The Pennsylvania State University, 201 Nursing Sciences Building, University Park, PA 16802, USA
* Corresponding author.
E-mail address: cmg35@psu.edu

Nurs Clin N Am 58 (2023) 1–10
https://doi.org/10.1016/j.cnur.2022.10.008
0029-6465/23/© 2022 Elsevier Inc. All rights reserved.

experienced this transition to online learning found concerns in regard to feeling iso-lated and missing hands-on experiences.[3]

The Ross and Carol Nese College of Nursing, The Pennsylvania State University, faced the same challenges as other schools of nursing in response to the pandemic and the abrupt transition to remote instruction. The college's simulation committee identified two main priorities when the pandemic began: (1) ensure that virtual clinical experiences were engaging, of high quality, and incorporated clinical judgment and (2) plan for the return to in-person instruction in the simulation laboratories as soon as it could be done safely.

Transition to Virtual Simulation

In response to the first priority, the committee reviewed literature on virtual simulation and identified a variety of resources such as virtual simulations that were available free online as well as products that were available from vendors. The committee deter-mined that it would be important to provide guidance to faculty in how to effectively incorporate these resources as they planned clinical replacement. A set of guidelines for virtual clinical were developed. The (INACSL) Standards of Best Practice: Simula-tion[SM6] were consulted in the development of these guidelines. Key points included in the guidelines were that all activities are based on measurable objectives, are participant-centered and driven by the objectives, and should include a synchronous debriefing with faculty. Synchronous debriefing has been identified as a best practice and was cited by students as an important component of maintaining engagement in their education.[3–5]

Planning for Return to In-Person Simulation

In response to the second priority, a task force was formed to plan for reopening simu-lation laboratories for Fall semester 2020. Multiple safety and infection control issues needed to be addressed including social distancing constraints, screening of students and faculty for signs and symptoms of COVID-19, cleaning and disinfecting protocols, obtaining necessary personal protective equipment (PPE) and establishing guidelines for its use, and how to effectively communicate guidelines to all faculty, staff, and stu-dents that would be using the laboratories.

PLANNING FOR SAFETY AND INFECTION CONTROL
Social Distancing Considerations

Rooms' capacities were limited to allow for social distancing in compliance with Cen-ters for Disease Control and university guidelines. This presented challenges in plan-ning laboratory activities. For example, typically a health assessment laboratory of up to ten students and their instructor would meet for a laboratory session or a clinical group of eight students would participate together in a simulation. These numbers had to be cut in half. As a result, we scheduled split laboratory sessions for health assessment. Instead of a 3-hour laboratory, half of the group would come for 90 mi-nutes, and then the other half of the group would come. The goal was to maximize hands on practice during these shortened sessions. A flipped classroom type approach was used. Students spent the time that they otherwise would have been in laboratory doing preparatory activities such as watching videos or completing writ-ten assignments. For simulation, we needed to be flexible. Larger classrooms that could accommodate an entire clinical group while maintaining social distancing were converted to debriefing spaces. Simulation rooms were limited to two-to-three learners. In addition to the flipped classroom approach, we either used video capture software to allow observers to view the simulation from the debriefing room or moved the simulator and other equipment into the room and had a "simulation in the round" approach.

Screening for Laboratory Entry

The university instituted routine, random COVID testing for all students and employees. In addition, the university had protocols for isolation and quarantine of individuals with COVID-19 or those who had been exposed. Because laboratory activities would require students to be less than 6 feet apart during skills practice or simulation, we instituted additional health screening procedures and the use of PPE. Fortunately, the university had developed a "symptom checker" app that was available to the university community. It would enable the user to answer questions about any possible symptoms or exposure to COVID-19. Students could show a screen indicating that they were good for entry when they arrived at the laboratory. We also obtained thermal scanning thermometers to check for fever before laboratory entry. Any temperature greater than 100.4° Fahrenheit would be criteria to deny entry. On entry to the laboratory, students would perform hand hygiene with soap and water for 20 seconds or use alcohol-based hand sanitizer.

Cleaning and Disinfecting Protocols

Cleaning and disinfecting surfaces and equipment in the simulation laboratory presented unique challenges. We had to ensure that decontamination without damaging expensive technology such as simulators and computers. There are multiple disinfecting products that kill COVID-19 but many of them were in short supply in 2020 or could damage the technology. Fortunately, 70% isopropyl alcohol can effectively disinfect for COVID-19 and can safely be used on the simulators. We obtained large volumes of it and had it available in spray bottles in each room. After every activity, surfaces and equipment were sprayed with the alcohol and allowed to dry. It is important that it not be wiped up before drying so it kills the virus. We had to be sure that students and faculty were instructed on this. Soft surfaces such as linens and curtains were another challenge, as they are not readily disinfected. We replaced linen sheets and gown with plastic that can be cleaned after each use and tied back privacy curtains.

Personal Protective Equipment

PPE was in short supply throughout 2020 and the priority was to ensure that direct care personnel had adequate PPE to do their jobs safely. At the onset of the pandemic, we donated our supply of PPE to local hospitals. By August 2020, N-95 masks were not available, but we were able to obtain an adequate supply of procedure masks, gloves, gowns, and face shields. The university instituted required masking in all buildings. When students in the laboratory would be within six feet of each other for laboratory practice or simulation, they donned gloves, gown, procedure masks, and face shields.

Communicating Guidelines

It was important to ensure that all faculty, staff, and students were fully informed of the COVID-19 guidelines for the simulation laboratories before the beginning of the school year in August 2020. To accomplish this, a learning module was developed in the university's learning management system that everyone accessing the simulation laboratory completed. The module included background on infection control principles, brief videos, and written materials on the use of PPE, cleaning and disinfecting, laboratory entry criteria, an attestation that the person agreed to abide by the guidelines, and a posttest to ensure knowledge of the guidelines. Users had to score 100% to pass the posttest and complete the module. Multiple attempts on the posttest were permitted to obtain the passing score. The module was embedded in a course at each level of the curriculum. Laboratory personnel could easily see who had completed the module.

Outcomes of Laboratory Reopening

We were able to successfully reopen our simulation laboratories to in-person learning in Fall 2020. Our infection control procedures were effective, as we are not aware of any COVID spread that resulted from laboratory activities. We had to be flexible in meeting student learning needs as access to clinical sites varied by course and location. We were able to meet the required clinical hours by using a combination of in-person clinical when available, face-to-face simulation and virtual simulation. We prioritized the use of laboratory to activities that would have the highest impact on student learning such as hand-on skills practice and high-fidelity simulations.

ADAPTATION OF LEARNING MODALITIES
Virtual Learning

Simulation-based learning experiences (SBLEs) provide students with an opportunity to develop skills to manage real-life clinical experiences. Virtual simulation learning experiences (VSLEs) are alternative strategies to consider if high-fidelity simulation is not feasible or cost-effective.[7] Foronda and colleagues[8] define virtual simulation as "clinical simulation offered on a computer, the Internet, or in a digital learning environment including single or multiuser platforms" (p. 27). There is support for using VSLE to improve knowledge, skill, performance, confidence, and clinical judgment.[9–12] During the early phase of the COVID-19 pandemic, our program quickly adapted our own simulation experiences to remote (VSLE) along with using multiple virtual simulation resources available online.

The VSLEs adapted from our own simulation scenarios were conducted synchronously over the Internet. Photos, video clips, and audio clips were embedded in a PowerPoint to replace the interaction with the manikin. Simulation sessions were held using Zoom technology. Assessment findings were presented when students asked. The cases unfolded in the same manner as in the laboratory. We wanted to maintain the focus on students independently interpreting patient data and making clinical judgments. Students evaluated the VSLEs using the same instrument used to evaluate high-fidelity simulations in the laboratory. The instrument asks students to rate the experience on a variety of factors including preparation to care for patients, realism, ability to recognize changes in conditions, learning of pathophysiology, pharmacology, and classroom information, assessment skills, teamwork, communication skills, and effectiveness of debriefing. Each item is rated on a 7-point scale from strongly disagree to strongly agree. Independent sample *t* tests were used to compare groups on one set of simulations that were converted to compare outcomes between the high-fidelity simulation and the VSLE. There were no significant differences on any item except that "developed better understanding of pathophysiology" was rated higher in the manikin group. The selected outcomes are detailed in **Table 1**.

Once our simulation laboratory space reopened, with social distancing restrictions, decisions were implemented to map out our learning options that included resuming face-to-face SBLEs scheduled in cohort with VSLEs. Considerations that were required to be addressed during this time included how to incorporate the ability to

Table 1
Student evaluation of selected learning outcomes

Learning Outcome	V-Sim		Manikin Sim		t(67)	P
	M	SD	M	SD		
The simulation was realistic	5.74	1.55	6.29	.90	1.711	.092
I am better prepared to care for patients	6.13	1.21	6.26	1.03	.461	.647
I am better understand the pathophysiology	6.53	.65	6.81	.40	2.200	.031
I am better understand the pharmacology	6.32	.87	6.65	.55	1.824	.073
I am more confident in decision-making	6.26	.92	6.26	.82	.024	.981
My assessment skills improved	5.87	1.30	6.29	.78	1.588	.117
I was changed to think like a nurse	6.61	.59	6.39	.75	1.338	.186
I am better prepared to use SBAR	6.63	.59	6.35	.75	1.711	.092
Debriefing provided time to reflect	6.54	.65	6.65	.55	.708	.481
Debriefing summarized key learning	6.61	.55	6.68	.54	.548	.586
Instructor helped me think critically	6.71	.46	6.74	.44	.286	.775

Note. Scale 1 = strongly disagree; 2 = disagree; 3 = somewhat disagree; 4 = neutral; 5 = somewhat agree; 6 = agree; 7 = strongly agree.
 Abbreviations: SBAR, *Situation, Background, Assessment, Recommendation.*

have students on site with clinical experiences in their agencies, clinical laboratory time for skills learning, and face-to-face SBLEs.

Scheduling for Learning Options

Limitation on the number of students who were able to participate in face-to-face SBLEs required shortening the time and number of students in simulation laboratory. This required a schedule that mapped out each experience and was accomplished by alternating face-to-face simulation with VSLEs and students in the clinical setting. The who, where, and then what needed to be considered in the scheduling process. The who involved staffing the simulation laboratory, faculty in on-site clinical, and faculty facilitating virtual clinical or simulation. Considerations for simulation included laboratory availability, the total number of students and facilitators permitted in each room, how long each simulation session required, and which simulations would be most effective in-person. Simulation experiences that could be as effective if delivered virtually were identified.

Resources

Faculty worked with simulation coordinators to plan their course and meet course objectives by identifying resources to design their experiences to meet clinical hours. Multiple resources were pulled together by our Simulation Committee to provide our faculty with a menu of options during the spring of 2020. These resources included Ryerson Virtual Healthcare Experience, Swift River Simulations, vSim for Nursing, and home-grown solutions such as developing PowerPoint presentations of our simulations for presentation virtually as described above.

Preparing for Simulation-Based Learning Experiences

Once our program returned to the simulation laboratory in the Fall of 2020, with social distancing limitations, course coordinators collaborated to map specific virtual experiences that would be incorporated into courses across the curriculum. Pre-briefing was modified to occur outside of the simulation laboratory using recordings of the pre-brief information in combination with pre-simulation assignments. Debriefing occurred with a synchronous meeting whether the simulation was held in-person or virtually.

The quick shift to the use of Zoom technology that occurred in the spring of 2020 integrated into a technology now used frequently in all courses. This has provided our program the ability to virtually debrief after participation in either a face-to-face or VSLE. Zoom has also provided the ability for peer interaction and collaboration facilitated by clinical faculty who are able to encourage student reflection and guide them in clinical thinking.

ENSURING QUALITY IN SIMULATION LEARNING EXPERIENCES
Planning the Activity

As a result of the pandemic, there are more resources available for selecting high-quality clinical replacement activities than before this unprecedented event in nursing education. This experience and knowledge have provided us with the ability to assess each learning situation and improve our decision-making skills in selecting the best quality replacement activities for students. Once possible options for types of replacement activities have been reviewed and narrowed down, the next step in ensuring the quality of the activity is for course coordinators and simulation faculty to work closely together to plan the activity. Many activities that had been implemented when the pandemic first began may no longer be available, or after evaluation of the activity, were found not to be the best option for ensuring a high-quality experience. When course faculty are tasked to modify clinical and simulation activities that have been in place and effective in learning for many years, it can be very overwhelming, especially when these changes to convert to an unfamiliar revised or remote learning may need to happen very quickly. To help alleviate some of the stress and anxiety over the situation, simulation faculty can assist course coordinators with analyzing needs and objectives for student learning and help to identify SBLEs that would best meet the objectives.

Ensuring Adherence to Standards of Best Practice

When moving from a face-to-face learning environment to a revised, remote, or virtual platform, the same standards for best practices still need to apply to simulation and clinical replacement activities. The guidelines for ensuring quality of simulations are available through the INACSL. INACSL Healthcare Simulation Standards of Best Practice (HSSOBP)[13] provides very clearly defined guidelines to follow for designing, implementing, and evaluating an SBLE. Even though some SBLEs may be predeveloped, as in a virtual simulation from a reputable company or as additional resources from a textbook, when integrating the activity into a course, the HSSOBP needs to be implemented to maintain a high-quality experience for students. Some of the standards we would apply in this situation are simulation design, outcomes and objectives, facilitation, debriefing, and participant evaluation.

Simulation design begins with a needs assessment to choose options for the learning activity. Faculty should ensure that the activity is equivalent in achieving the knowledge, skills, and behaviors as the activity that it is replacing. The conclusions from the needs assessment will direct the development of the learning objectives to enable students to reach the intended outcomes of the replacement activity. The objectives should be specific, measurable, achievable, realistic, and time-phased

(SMART objectives).[13] Collaboration between simulation faculty and course faculty is a valuable resource in ensuring alignment of the needs and objectives. It is important to consider not just the title of the activity, but how the content of the activity may need to be modified to meet the course needs.

Facilitation is the next step of the process and must include a necessary pre-brief and elements such as ensuring that appropriate cues are incorporated into the activity. The pre-brief is an essential component of the facilitation process for simulation activities. This should provide students with expectations and patient information for the activity as well as an orientation to the simulation environment is it virtual or face to face.[13] Faculty should provide materials and resources to prepare the students to be successful in achieving intended outcomes of the replacement activity. If students are not given the appropriate information to prepare for the activity, then they may tend to get caught up in focusing on irrelevant tasks, skills, or materials within the activity that lead them away from their intended objectives. For predeveloped, revised, or modified simulation and clinical replacement activities, the simulation faculty can assist the course coordinator in designing a pre-brief specifically for that activity, and then help to evaluate if the pre-brief contains the necessary information for the students to achieve their objectives.

Debriefing, while not included in many predeveloped activities, it is critical for reflecting and processing new knowledge with peers, self, and the instructor. It is important to remember that the facilitation of the simulation does not end with the students' completion of the activity. A critical part of learning with clinical or simulations is the teamwork experiences where they give and receive feedback. This is essential in beginning to think like a nurse. The post-conference after the clinical experience and the debriefing session after the simulation experience are important for development of clinical judgment for students through peer and self-reflection as well as instructor feedback. It is important to continue to include this key teaching tool with all replacement activities, whether it is a predeveloped type of simulation or a redesigned simulation activity. As many of the predeveloped types of replacement activities may contain some form of post-activity questions or discussion points, simulation faculty can assist the course faculty in revising the questions to produce a meaningful debriefing session. If course faculty are using a modified or redesigned clinical simulation experience, simulation faculty are a great resource to assist course faculty in planning and designing the debriefing session. There are several effective theory-based debriefing models that simulation faculty use to guide the session toward high-quality feedback and self-reflection that meet the intended objectives and outcomes of the activity. Using these strategies, simulation faculty can design some type of a rubric, checklist, or other tool to assist in directing the debriefing for course faculty and to increase student engagement in the session. Finally, the activity needs to include a plan for participant evaluation. The evaluation plan is developed to ensure it will measure the achievement of learning objectives. The steps for planning and developing effective clinical learning replacement are illustrated in **Fig. 1**.

EVALUATING SIMULATION EXPERIENCES
Importance of Evaluation

With the rapid adoption of virtual simulation at the onset of the pandemic, the environment of face-to-face simulation changes dramatically. Evaluating the effectiveness of simulation experiences, whether virtual or face to face, is imperative to assess the quality of simulation experiences. The use of valid and reliable instruments to collect

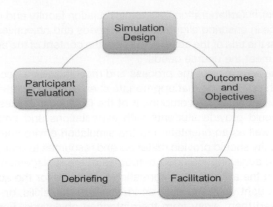

Fig. 1. Process for developing clinical replacement activities.

student feedback regarding satisfaction with simulation modalities provides information to make appropriate changes as necessary. A variety of evaluation instruments should be used throughout your simulation program to reflect your vision and integration of simulation in your curriculum.

The model below (**Fig. 2**) reflects the cycle of building your simulation evaluation program.

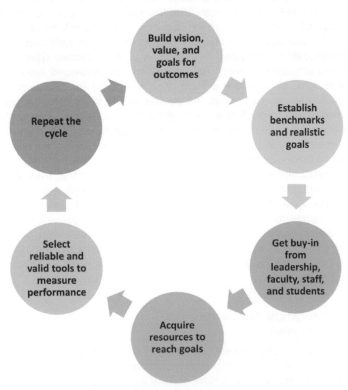

Fig. 2. Evaluation model for simulation.

Tools to Evaluate Simulation

There are many valid and reliable tools to evaluate simulation. One that is widely used is the SET-M which is designed for evaluating simulation scenario and is useful for evaluating learner's perception of how effective the simulation was toward meeting their learning needs.[14] Our simulation program uses this tool with the example of student feedback provided in **Table 1**.

The CLECS 2.0[15] is an instrument ideal for our pandemic environment because it measures student perceptions of how well their learning needs are met in three environments: traditional clinical environment, face-to-face simulated clinical environment, and screen-based simulation or virtual simulation. The utilization of this instrument can identify if facilitators are meeting the learning needs of students, identify clinical experiences for areas requiring improvement, and also identify curricular gaps.

Integrative Learning Evaluation

Integrative learning is the process of making connections among concepts and experiences so that information and skills can be applied to novel and complex issues or challenges. This is apparent as we use the concept of Bloom's taxonomy to build our simulation program from simple to complex scenarios.

Evaluating integrative learning can include pretesting and posttesting questions regarding a simulation experience, written examination questions on course examinations, and student self-evaluations regarding meeting simulation, course, and program outcomes. The curriculum could also build in a repeat of a simulation at a higher level that includes more complex issues, using a deliberate practice model.

POST-COVID: A TIME FOR NEW BEGINNINGS

The pandemic challenged nursing education to adopt the delivery of simulation laboratory experiences including both clinical skills and SBLEs. Simulation educators had to rethink and reconfigure how simulation curriculum was delivered. These adaptations were necessary in order to create clinical opportunities for our students. As we emerge from the pandemic into a new era now is the time for reflection on the variety of resources and scheduling modifications implemented. This presents the question as to which innovative adaptations were effective and could be now be incorporated into a simulation curriculum.

Simulation educators need to consider which of the adopted resources maintain best practice for simulation while providing the simulation laboratory with cost-effective and time-saving experiences. The innovative virtual experiences that provided students with additional opportunities to develop their clinical skills, therefore, need to be evaluated for how to be best implemented along with face-to-face SBLEs. We have no idea if another event may cause disruption in our simulation programs but we are now prepared to face that and to use the resources that emerged to create a new beginning for simulation programs.

CLINICS CARE POINTS

- Incorporate synchronous debriefing for virtual simulations
- Evaluate all simulations using validated instruments
- Screen participants for s/s of COVID on entry to the laboratory

- Have adequate personal protective equipment available
- Disinfect surfaces and equipment with 70% isopropyl alcohol.
- Follow Healthcare Standards of Best Practices regardless of simulation methodology.

DISCLOSURE

The authors have no financial or commercial conflicts of interest to disclose and received no funding for this project.

REFERENCES

1. Cucinotta D, Vanelli M. WHO Declares COVID-19 a Pandemic. Acta Biomed 2020;91(1):157–60.
2. Leaver CA, Stanley JM, Veenema TG. Impact of the COVID-19 pandemic on the future of nursing education. Acad Med 2022;97(35):S82–9.
3. Michel A, Ryan N, Mattheus D, et al. Undergraduate nursing students' perceptions on nursing education during the 2020 COVID-19 pandemic: A national sample. Nurs Outlook 2021;69:903–12.
4. Esposito CP, Sullivan K. Maintaining clinical continuity through virtual simulation during the COVID-19 pandemic. J Nurs Educ 2020;59(9):522–5.
5. Shea KL, Rovera EJ. Preparing for the COVID-19 pandemic and its impact on a nursing simulation curriculum. J Nurs Educ 2021;60(1):52–5.
6. INACSL Standards Committee. INACSL Standards of Best Practice: Simulation^{SM}. Clin Simulation Nurs 2016;12:S1–50.
7. Verkuyl M, Atack L, Mastrilli P, et al. Virtual gaming to develop students' pediatric nursing skills: A usability test. Nurse Educ Today 2016;46:81–5.
8. Foronda CL, Swoboda SM, Henry MN, et al. Student preferences and perceptions of learning from vSim for nursing. Nurse Educ Pract 2018;33:27–32.
9. Foronda CL, Fernandez-Burgos M, Nadeau C, et al. Virtual simulation in nursing education: A systematic review spanning 1996 to 2018. Simulation Healthc 2020; 15(1):46–54.
10. Liaw SY, Chan SW, Chen F, et al. Comparison of virtual patient simulation with mannequin-based simulation for improving clinical performance in assessing and managing clinical deterioration: Randomized controlled trial. JMIR Med Educ 2014;16(9):e214.
11. Padilha JM, Machado PP, Ribeiro A, et al. Clinical virtual simulation in nursing education: A randomized controlled trial. JMIR Med Educ 2019;21(3):e11529.
12. Shin H, Rim D, Kim H, et al. Educational characteristics of virtual simulation in nursing: An integrative review. Clin Simulation Nurs 2019;37:18–28.
13. INACSL Standards Committee. Healthcare Simulation Standards of Best Practice^{TM}. Clin Simulation Nurs 2021;58:1–66.
14. Leighton K, Ravert P, Mudra V, et al. Simulation Effectiveness Tool-Modified. 2018. https://sites.google.com/view/evaluatinghealthcaresimulation/set-m. [Accessed 21 June 2022].
15. Leighton K. CLECS 2.0. 2019. https://sites.google.com/view/evaluatinghealthcaresimulation/clecs/clecs-2-0. [Accessed 21 June 2022].

Mobilizing the Community to Implement Mass Coronavirus Disease-2019 Vaccination Clinics

The Power of Free and Charitable Clinics

Kristi Mattzela, MSW, LSW[a], Cheryl Jo White, RN[a],
Lori A. Francis, PhD[b],*

KEYWORDS

- COVID-19 vaccine • Free and charitable clinics • Mass vaccination
- Rural health care

KEY POINTS

- A small, community clinic provided more than 44,000 coronavirus disease-2019vaccine doses in a semirural community.
- Mass vaccination clinics can be implemented by small health care systems using a volunteer model.
- Given their volunteer model, free and charitable clinics are well poised to implement mass vaccination clinics.
- Community clinics, as a trusted source of health care, have the power to address vaccine hesitancy in the community.

INTRODUCTION

Coronavirus disease-2019 (COVID-19) vaccines have been shown to be efficacious in significantly reducing severe acute respiratory syndrome coronavirus 2 (SARS-CoV-2) infection, severe illness, hospitalization, and mortality, particularly among individuals who receive at least two doses.[1] The vaccines were developed rapidly, in less than 12 months,[2] despite most vaccines taking up to 10 years or more to be developed. This accelerated vaccine development pace presented several challenges for health

[a] Centre Volunteers in Medicine, State College, 2520 Green Tech Drive, Suite D, State College, PA 16803, USA; [b] Department of Biobehavioral Health, The Pennsylvania State University, 219 Biobehavioral Health Building, University Park, PA 16802, USA
* Corresponding author.
E-mail address: lfrancis@psu.edu
Twitter: @CentreCVIM (K.M.); @CentreCVIM (C.J.W.)

Nurs Clin N Am 58 (2023) 11–23
https://doi.org/10.1016/j.cnur.2022.10.001
0029-6465/23/© 2022 Elsevier Inc. All rights reserved.

care systems and local public health agencies, including difficulties acquiring the vaccine, difficulties securing adequate space and equipment to store vaccine doses, difficulties mobilizing health care systems to vaccinate individuals in large volumes, and vaccine hesitancy given uncertainty about the short- and long-term effects of the vaccine.[3-5]

Rural areas are faced with unique challenges due to geographic isolation and greater levels of vaccine hesitancy.[6-8] A national US study of adults found that rural respondents were more likely to report feeling that the COVID-19 vaccine was unsafe.[9] Using the use of mass vaccination hubs within communities has been shown to increase vaccination reach.[10] Furthermore, community clinics can play an important role in vaccination efforts within communities, given that (1) they often rely on a volunteer model of care, which is crucial for mass vaccination efforts, and (2) they may be serving individuals at higher risk for vaccine hesitancy. The purpose of this article is to describe the design and implementation of large-scale, mass vaccination clinics implemented by a small community clinic in a semirural area in Pennsylvania.

METHODS
Clinic History

Centre Volunteers in Medicine (CVIM) is a free and charitable community clinic that provides medical care, dental care, case management, behavioral health services, and medication assistance to those without health insurance and whose household income is at or less than 250% of the federal poverty level. CVIM serves those living or working in Centre County, PA. In addition to a small paid staff, the clinic is mainly staffed by physicians, nurses, dentists, pharmacists, social workers, and other licensed clinicians who volunteer their time to provide care to patients. In addition, referrals are provided to specialists and social service agencies as necessary. In the fiscal year 2018 to 19, CVIM served a total of 483 medical and 632 dental patients, with a total of 1427 and 2355 medical and dental visits, respectively.

The first Volunteers in Medicine Clinic opened in Hilton Head, South Carolina, in 1991. Since then, many additional clinics have begun serving the uninsured and underinsured nationwide. The clinics function on volunteers who provide a caring and compassionate medical home for those who do not qualify for medical assistance and/or are working without health care benefits. Efforts to establish a Volunteers in Medicine Clinic in Centre County, PA, began in February 2001 when a group of local citizens met to address health care needs in the Centre Region. CVIM was incorporated as a nonprofit organization on June 12, 2001. In February 2003, CVIM opened its doors to patients seeking medical care. Based on data provided in a 2019 Community Health Needs Assessment report[11] from a local health care system, 11 townships served by CVIM are considered medically-underserved areas, and two major towns served by CVIM are considered Health care Professional Shortage Areas.

Coronavirus Disease-2019 Vaccine Clinic Timeline

Owing to the rapid COVID-19 vaccine development timeline, efforts to mobilize for mass public vaccination had to occur at an accelerated speed. CVIM applied to be a vaccine recipient in the State of Pennsylvania in November 2020. Vaccine storage requirements and preparation procedures were researched, and staff began writing standard operating procedures and policies, in addition to completing several trainings. A total of 3 CVIM staff were trained to manage vaccine doses. In addition, a freezer was purchased for vaccine storage. CVIM's approval to become a vaccine recipient was granted in December 2020, and vaccine orders began to be placed the same month.

The COVID-19 vaccine became available to the public on December 11, 2020, but only to special populations, including first responders, health care workers, essential workers, older adults ($\geq$65 years), and adults with specific underlying medical conditions, such as cancer, diabetes, and obesity. By April 2021, the vaccine was available to all US adults ($\geq$18 years), although the vaccine shortage limited the number of doses that could successfully be administered within a 7-day period. CVIM's first shipment of 100 Moderna vaccine doses arrived on January 13, 2021, and efforts were focused on vaccinating clinic volunteers $\geq$65 years.

In January 2021, CVIM, the local hospital, pharmacies, and a small apothecary were the only entities that were vaccine recipients. Given staffing and scheduling restraints, we estimated that it would take nearly 2 years to vaccinate the county. Based on data from the US Census Bureau (www.census.gov/quickfacts/centrecountypennsylvania), the Centre County, PA population size was estimated to be 158,172 in April 2020, and some entities could only schedule a maximum of 10 vaccinations/d. Given how smoothly the initial, in-house volunteer vaccine clinics operated, CVIM recognized their capacity to address the vaccine demand and needs of the larger community, and they began to mobilize to offer mass vaccination clinics. CVIM began administering the Moderna vaccine in January 2021, the Pfizer vaccine in February 2021 and the Johnson & Johnson single-dose vaccines in April 2021; all vaccines were offered after April 2021.

"Super Saturday" Mass Vaccination Clinic Planning and Mobilization

Word that CVIM was a vaccine recipient began to spread rapidly throughout the county, and residents began to contact CVIM for vaccine appointments before additional vaccine doses were available. A waiting list was created and grew exponentially (>10,000 individuals). This provided unequivocal evidence that the demand for the vaccine was great. CVIM saw an opportunity to address this demand, and given its volunteer model, they determined that they would be able to mobilize volunteers on a large scale to meet the demand. In addition, given the burden that the local hospital and other health care entities were experiencing as a result of the pandemic, including health care professional shortages, and staff who were overstretched and experiencing burnout, CVIM was committed to lessening the burden on community providers who had supported them in the past. Most importantly, CVIM was committed to playing an active role in public health efforts to end COVID-19. CVIM had the bandwidth and energy available for this important purpose. As such, efforts to develop and implement mass COVID-19 vaccination clinics began in January 2021. Plans were made to offer the mass vaccination clinics on Saturdays, and to name them "Super Saturday Clinics."

Space and room capacity. Since 2008, CVIM has been housed in a building with 6217 square feet of clinic space, including a waiting/check-in area that can seat up to 10 patients (five during COVID to allow for social distancing), with an adjoining bathroom, six examination rooms, three case management rooms, and four dental operatories. Given that CVIM was continuing to see medical, dental, and behavioral health patients as part of its normal operations, it would have been difficult to offer a mass vaccination clinic in-house. With the space, staffing, and schedule constraints, the maximum number of vaccination that could have been administered in the in-house clinic was 150/d. CVIM administrators met with an administrator in the local area school district in January 2021, and we were invited to use a local school for mass vaccine clinics (**Figs. 1** and **2**). Available for use were the lobby for check-in, two classrooms for preparation of vaccine doses and data entry, the cafeteria for completion

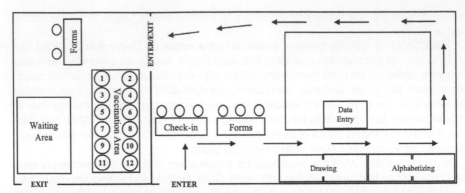

Fig. 1. Example layout and traffic flow for the "Super Saturday" mass vaccination clinics in the school locations for individuals 12+ years. This figure is not to scale.

of forms, and the gymnasium for vaccine administration and post-vaccine waiting areas. In addition, CVIM partnered with a local university, other nearby school districts, and local YMCA locations in neighboring communities to provide traveling mass vaccine clinics.

In October 2021, CVIM purchased a new building with 10,980 square feet of clinic space, which added a larger check-in area and additional space in the waiting area with seating for up to 80 patients. This location also added 15 private examination rooms, and additional space for storing, preparing, and administering vaccines (**Fig. 3**). CVIM began using the new building for vaccination clinics while plans were

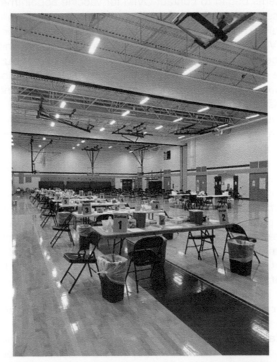

Fig. 2. Image of the layout of the vaccine clinics held in the local middle school gymnasium.

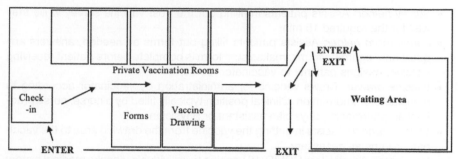

Fig. 3. Layout and traffic flow for the mass vaccination clinics for children ages 5 to 11 years. This figure is not to scale.

underway to renovate the building for a new clinic (eg, design, permitting, and zoning). In addition, school buildings were no longer available once students returned in the Fall of 2021.

Vaccine storage requirements and capacity. CVIM initially only provided the Moderna vaccine given smaller shipments (100 doses/tray) and required storage between −58°F and 5°F. The Pfizer vaccine shipped in larger quantities of 1170 doses/tray (6 doses in 195 multidose vials), and required storage between −130°F and −76°F before mixing, necessitating the need for an ultra-cold freezer. The Pennsylvania Department of Health contacted CVIM to request that they accept the Pfizer vaccine. At the time, CVIM was receiving 300 to 500 doses of Moderna vaccine per shipment and was requesting substantially more. CVIM agreed to take a tray of Pfizer 1170 vaccine doses and began mobilizing to offer a mass vaccine clinic to extend the dosing within 7 days, which was the time frame required by the Pennsylvania Department of Health. Once the vaccine doses were thawed and diluted, they could be stored in the refrigerator or at room temperature (35° to 77° F) and had to be used within 6 h. As such, clinic staff and volunteers needed to be trained on transferring and handling vaccines.

Staffing and training. For the smaller, in-house clinics, only three clinic staff members were needed for implementation (staff nurse, Clinical Services Director and Clinical Pharmacist). All clinic staff were paid staff with prior experience preparing and/or administering vaccines. However, due to the stringent requirements for transferring and handling vaccines, these clinic staff underwent extensive training on administering COVID-19 vaccines. The Centers for Disease Control and Prevention (CDC) held mandatory training for vaccine providers, and CVIM also held training for staff on internal protocols and procedures. To scale up for mass vaccination clinics, we determined that the following positions would be needed at each clinic:

- *Parking and external traffic flow:* Directed patients to clinic, monitored parking, directed people to open parking spots; directed exit out of parking lot. Often volunteers from the local police and fire departments.
- *Door monitor:* Stands outside and admits patients at the time of their time of appointment. Manages the flow of walk-in traffic.
- *Internal traffic flow:* Directs patients to the check-in area, the room to complete forms, the waiting room and the exit.
- *Check-in:* Ensures patient is eligible for vaccine. Provides correct form on clipboard with COVID-19 vaccine fact sheet. Checks name off of list (for scheduled vaccines) or completes information on walk-in sheet.

- *Survey helper*: Assists patients in filling out the post vaccine survey while they wait for the required 15 min.
- *Forms room helper*: Assists patients filling out forms as needed, answers any questions regarding forms, makes sure form is complete before patient receiving vaccine. Assigns patients to vaccinator rooms.
- *Vaccine drawer*: Draws vaccine for administration by vaccinator according to manufacturer information. Clinical position typically filled by a nurse, nurse practitioner, pharmacist, physician assistant or physician.
- *Vaccine runner*: Assists in getting the vaccine from the drawing area to the vaccinator rooms as necessary.
- *Vaccinator*: Administers COVID-19 vaccine to individuals, checks medical history and allergies before administering the vaccine. Clinical position typically filled by a nurse, nurse practitioner, pharmacist, physician assistant or physician.
- *Clipboard/form runner*: Collects clipboards from vaccinators, takes completed forms to data entry, cleans and sanitized clipboards and pens, rebuilds clipboards with new forms. Collects pens and returns to check in area.
- *Data entry:* Enter vaccination data into the state system.
- *Watcher*: Monitors and remains with patients for 15 min after vaccine is given to watch for adverse reactions. Alerts medical staff if necessary.
- *Emergency medical technician*: Oversees people waiting the 15 min period following the injection to assure no adverse effects. Offers support and care to anyone needing it. Must be licensed/certified.
- *Lunch volunteer/miscellaneous:* Assure there were drinks and snacks available for the volunteers, along with many other varied tasks that arose

Recruiting, training and managing volunteers. There was no shortage of health care workers that contacted CVIM to volunteer to help with vaccination efforts. Approximately 150 volunteers were needed for each "Super Saturday" clinic, and 480 total volunteers committed their time. Clinicians included doctors and nurses, both retired and still working. Clinicians noted that they wanted to help end this pandemic and be part of the solution, rather than simply taking care of patients who were dying from COVID-19. In addition to volunteers who reached out to serve, CVIM also sent out requests for volunteers through their extensive network of current and past clinic volunteers. Social media posts were also used for recruitment of volunteers. Depending on the volunteer position, training occurred on site approximately 1 h before the vaccination clinic opened. Vaccinators were trained on required paperwork and were responsible for completing a training on the COVID-19 vaccine types and administration on their own. There was a mandatory vaccinator training for retired individuals to ensure that they were aware of vaccination procedures and best practices. Vaccine drawers were required to watch a training video, after which they were observed while drawing vaccine to assure proper technique. The Clinical Nurse in charge was responsible for training all vaccinator volunteers on the procedures for each clinic. The clinical pharmacist was responsible for training vaccine drawers. Extensive training was provided until CVIM staff were confident that the volunteers were proficient with their assigned task. Several CVIM staff coordinators managed volunteer sign-ups and schedules, and directed volunteers to their various stations upon arrival at the vaccine clinic.

Advertising to the public. With each important milestone in vaccine development and availability, CVIM created social media posts on Facebook and Instagram. Estimated reach, likes and shares were measured. In addition, the number of clicks on embedded links was measured and used as a measure of vaccine uptake.

Vaccination Clinic Implementation

Adjustments were made to the formula for in-house vaccinations (3 vaccinations every 5 min) to account for the substantially larger space, and an exponentially larger amount of people. Using a conservative estimate, it was determined that each vaccinator would be able to vaccinate 1 individual every 5 min, for and approximation of 12 vaccination per hour, per vaccinator. A total of 24 vaccine drawers and 24 vaccinators were scheduled for the mass vaccination clinics. All CDC guidelines and protocols for storing, handling, transporting, preparing, and administering COVID-19 vaccines were followed (see www.cdc.gov/vaccines/hcp/admin/storage/toolkit/index.html). Vaccine doses were stored at CVIM before transport to the clinic. CVIM's clinical pharmacist was responsible for quality control and fidelity of all protocols and procedures, including thawing doses, monitoring temperatures, packing the transport container, and transporting vaccine doses to clinic locations. Refrigerators were often available for use at vaccine clinic locations to maintain consistent temperatures. Doses were prepped 1 h before the clinic. Vaccine drawers would draw each vial placing the doses from that vial in a bag labeled with the date/time it was drawn, and the time it expired. The vial was also placed in the bag so that vaccinators could see which vial the vaccine came from. A color coding system (lids, labels, forms) was used to identify Pfizer, Moderna, and Johnson & Johnson vaccines, and additional color coding was used for children's doses.

Vaccine stations were set up by a clinical nurse and supplies were stocked accordingly. Check-in tables were set up with printed schedules, clipboards and pens before patients arriving. Data entry set up their computers and their baskets containing completed and uncompleted forms. The EMT would set up a station with Epi Pens, juice and other equipment that may be needed if anyone had an adverse reaction to the vaccine. Chairs were set up in the forms completion area and the post-vaccination watching/waiting area. In school districts, janitorial staff (paid by the school district) assisted with setup, and school administrators volunteers their time to help manage the flow and assist with accessibility needs. The Clinical Director would walk through to assure that every area was ready before the start of the clinic.

Door monitors were stationed outside to greet patients as they arrived; they informed patients of what to expect and how the clinic ran. Vaccine appointments were scheduled in 5-min blocks (between 12 and 24 patients per block), and only those individuals with an appointment were permitted to enter the building during that time. This allowed for adequate social distancing and an orderly check-in process. Individuals were held outside of the building until their appointment time was called by the door monitor. During the check-in process, patients' vaccine eligibility was verified, and they would either receive their vaccine card for the first dose, or have their card checked for the second dose/booster. Individuals were then directed to the next station through a one-way hallway, where they would receive a health and consent form. One-way traffic flow and limited time waiting indoors helped to limit exposures and contact between individuals. Patients were seated in the vaccination waiting area to complete their forms, after which the forms were checked by a Survey Helper who also answered any questions. A Forms Room Helper then directed the patient to a shared vaccination station (two stations/table). After the patient was seated, the vaccinator reviewed the individual's health history and confirmed which vaccine they wanted to receive. Once the vaccination dose was administered, the patient was then directed to the waiting area where they would be asked to remain for 15 min. At this point, the Watcher would monitor and check-in with individuals to watch for any adverse reactions. The Emergency Medical Technician was nearby the waiting area to address any medical concerns that arose. All seating areas, pens and clipboard were sanitized at each station after each individual left that station.

The models and formulas used to implement vaccine clinics in the local clinic were also used to plan for vaccine clinics offered in other locations and throughout the county. Once it was determined how many vaccinators could fit into a space, while maintaining social distance, the planned clinics were either scaled up or down. This model proved to be very flexible and afforded us the ability to travel all over the county. Standard operating procedures for safe handling and transporting allowed us to maintain vaccine temperatures on longer distances.

Once approval to begin vaccinations for children ages 5 to 11 years was received, pediatric vaccination clinics were offered at CVIM's new clinic location (**Fig. 4**). CVIM had not initially planned to vaccinate this age group; however, local pediatricians requested assistance with their vaccination efforts. All procedures outlined for the school location above were followed for the pediatric clinics; however, individual vaccination stations were offered in private rooms. In addition, sidewalks approaching the building and entrances were decorated with welcoming messages, and volunteers were dressed in costumes at the entrance and at each station (vaccinators were not dressed in costumes). After receiving their vaccination, children were able to choose their own bandage and sticker, and child-friendly coloring and activity pages were provided in the waiting area (see **Fig. 4**). Children were invited to hang their decorated pictures in the clinic hallway.

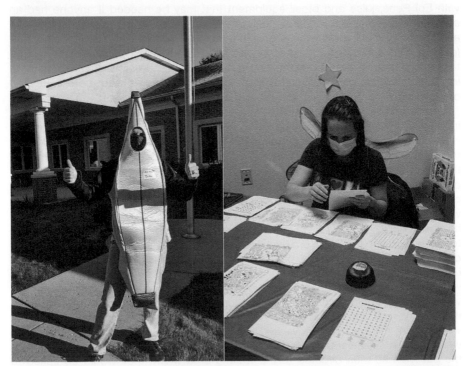

Fig. 4. Images of a greeter stationed outside of the pediatric clinic (pictured left) and the post-vaccination activity station (pictured right).

RESULTS

A total of 172 vaccine clinics and 44,634 vaccine doses were administered between January 2021 and June 2022. A total of 30 CVIM staff and volunteers were vaccinated at the initial clinic, and an additional 70 CVIM volunteers were vaccinated to expend the remaining vaccine doses. A maximum of 150 doses were administered at the CVIM clinic, before mass vaccination clinics were offered. **Fig. 5** provides a visual of the number of doses administered by month, along with the cumulative tallies. Approximately 2300 to 2400 individuals were vaccinated, on average, during a mass vaccination clinic, using 24 vaccinators and 24 vaccine drawers. Typically, approximately 50% ($n = 1200$) of these were first doses and 1200 were second doses. Of the 44,634 vaccine doses administered, 75.2% ($n = 33,574$) were among adults $\geq$ 19 years, 16.4% ($n = 7310$) were among youth ages 11 to 18 years, and 8.4% ($n = 3750$) were among children ages 5 to 11 years. No serious vaccine-related adverse reactions/events were reported. A few patients reported minor reactions, included soreness, rash or swelling at the injection site, lightheadedness, or feeling anxious about the injection; these reactions were not recorded. Emergency medical services were needed for one patient who experienced a syncopal episode that was unrelated to the vaccine.

As shown in **Fig. 5**, the demand for vaccinations was waning by the end of June 2021. This allowed the clinic's focus to shift to outreach to more rural communities. With the approval of boosters in August and September 2021, the demand for vaccines once again increased. A similar pattern was seen when vaccines were approved for use in children ages 5 to 11 years in November 2021.

Social media outreach and vaccine uptake. A total of 106 social media announcements were posted between January 2021 and June 2022 related to COVID-19, the availability of vaccines, and information about signing up for appointments. Several posts were also designed to demystify the vaccine and provide education based on scientific evidence. The reach of posts ranged from 32 individuals (Instagram, link to

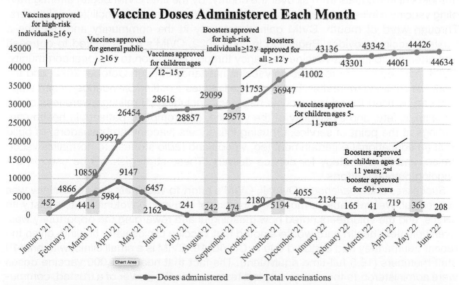

Fig. 5. Number of monthly vaccine doses administered, along with the cumulative totals over time. Important vaccine development dates are superimposed.

education on booster shots, May 2022) to 4514 (Facebook, link to schedule an appointment, December 2021). Clicks on embedded links ranged from 0 to 837 (Facebook, link to schedule an appointment, April 2021), and posts were shared between 0 and 61 times; the highest shares were from Facebook, with a link to schedule an appointment in April 2021.

Community Reaction

Although vaccines were provided for free, it was estimated that the true cost of providing a vaccine was $5 per vaccine. Thus, as a free and charitable clinic, donations were used to offset the cost of providing vaccinations. An unexpected windfall of financial donations poured in as a result of CVIM's mass vaccination clinics. It is likely that a large majority of individuals who attended the clinics were not familiar with CVIM until vaccination clinics were offered. In 2019 and 2020, CVIM saw an increase in their donor base of 330 and 409 new donors, respectively. During 2021, when vaccination clinics were offered, there were 1090 new donors, which represents nearly a 300% increase in new donors.

DISCUSSION

The overall success of CVIM's mass vaccination clinics highlights the promise of community clinics to respond to public health emergencies and address community vaccination needs. Given the volunteer model used by free and charitable clinics similar to CVIM, such entities are uniquely poised to quickly mobilize volunteers. Hasan and colleagues[10] recommend engaging the community in mass vaccination efforts, including volunteer inclusion and training and the use of social media platforms to share information.

Once CVIM's mass vaccination clinic location was switched to a local school, neighboring school districts began requesting mass vaccination clinics at their locations. This proved to be very successful and CVIM was able to continue vaccinating large numbers of individuals from all over the county. By the time CVIM began offering traveling vaccine clinics, they had attracted nearly 500 clinical and nonclinical volunteers. Through word of mouth, CVIM gained notoriety in the community and became a trusted vaccine provider. Beginning in June 2022, CVIM's focus shifted to outreach and attempts to impact vaccine hesitancy through education to the local community. CVIM received a grant to focus on vaccine hesitancy through October 2022, and the work will continue thereafter. Evans and colleagues[12] outline 5 evidence-based steps that can be used to reduce vaccine hesitancy, including (1) raising awareness of the benefits, safety, and availability of the vaccine, (2) prompting patients in health care settings at the point of service, (3) using influencers (vaccine ambassadors) to build trust (4) educational entertainment (eg, videos and radio stories), to normalize vaccination, and (5) a strategy for service delivery. These strategies will be used in our ongoing outreach efforts.

Successes and challenges. Overall, CVIM's effort to vaccinate the community was successful. We were able to mobilize hundreds of community volunteers to assist with clinics, and the volunteers noted how meaningful and rewarding the opportunity was. Even volunteer health care workers noted that vaccine clinics were healing, given the recent trauma they had endured due to COVID-19. CVIM is a small clinic, with only 19 staff members (16.5 full-time equivalent). The fact that nearly 45,000 vaccine doses were administered to the community is a testament to the power of a trusted, community clinic's ability to garner tremendous support from the community to respond to public health emergencies. Patients attending vaccination clinics consistently shared that the clinic was welcoming and volunteers were kind. This may have increased the likelihood that patients would return for second vaccines and boosters. CVIM created a fun and child-friendly atmosphere for the pediatric clinics. Parents noted that the clinics were efficient, and that staff and volunteers made their children feel comfortable. A review by Chambers and colleagues[13] showed that distraction techniques can be efficacious at reducing children's distress during immunizations. Although volunteers in costumes were not a method that was specifically addressed in this review, it is likely that this served as a distraction technique. Many children reported to their parents that they wanted to receive all of their vaccines from CVIM due to the pleasant experience we created.

The vaccine implementation work was not without challenges. Major challenges were experienced in providing vaccines, mainly due to the initial application process and lack of vaccine supply. At times, the waiting lists being maintained reached upwards of 10,000 individuals, which was a difficult task to manage and coordinate. Given the potential for waste of unused doses, lists of eligible individuals who could be reached on short notice were maintained. Within a few weeks, over 10,000 individuals were on a waiting list. Each person would need to be called and individually scheduled for clinics. CVIM was the only local entity scheduling appointments by phone. We were determined to make vaccinations available to those who did not have access to email, and this was critical for seniors in the community. This process was very time intensive, and a group of volunteers was mobilized to help with this effort. It is estimated that less than 3% of doses were wasted. When vaccinating in mass quantities, tracking vaccine lot numbers can be challenging. It was important to assure that the correct information was recorded on an individual's vaccine card. The logistics of efficient tracking required detail-oriented staff with excellent organizational and communication skills. Overall, the logistics of operating a mass vaccination clinic were significant. Having a highly efficient, organized and responsible team was critical to the success.

SUMMARY

Community clinics can play a vital role in local community vaccination efforts to address and improve patient outcomes. Given current community partnerships with hospitals, health care systems, social service agencies, and other local entities (eg, schools, churches, and other charitable organizations), community clinics can leverage local networks, including a large volunteer base, to respond to public health emergencies like COVID-19.

CLINICS CARE POINTS

- Community clinics can effectively and efficiently respond to public health efforts to increase vaccination reach
- Engaging the community in responses to public health emergencies can increase the success of vaccination clinics
- The process of applying to become a vaccine site can be arduous and cumbersome. It is recommended that clinics connect with the local Department of Health for assistance and support.
- When asked, the health care community will step up and help in a crisis and do so willingly and selflessly to help their community.

- Community partners are critical to success with a project like this. It would not have been possible without our community partners, like local school districts and universities.
- Creating an initiative like this requires strong leadership, planning, organization, and a well-running team who can handle stress and who can also take on creating structure in their area.
- If you focus on patients and the need, the rest will fall into place.

DISCLOSURE

The authors have nothing to disclose.

ACKNOWLEDGMENTS

Center Volunteers in Medicine would like to thank all of the volunteers and donors who helped to make our COVID-19 vaccination efforts a major success. The authors are eternally grateful for your selflessness, and your commitment to ending the COVID-19 pandemic.

REFERENCES

1. Dagan N, Barda N, Kepten E, et al. BNT162b2 mRNA Covid-19 Vaccine in a Nationwide Mass Vaccination Setting. N Engl J Med 2021;384(15):1412–23.
2. Wouters OJ, Shadlen KC, Salcher-Konrad M, et al. Challenges in ensuring global access to COVID-19 vaccines: production, affordability, allocation, and deployment. Lancet 2021;397(10278):1023–34.
3. Alam ST, Ahmed S, Ali SM, et al. Challenges to COVID-19 vaccine supply chain: Implications for sustainable development goals. Int J Prod Econ 2021;239: 108193.
4. Kim D, Pekgün P, Yildirim İ, et al. Resource allocation for different types of vaccines against COVID-19: Tradeoffs and synergies between efficacy and reach. Vaccine 2021;39(47):6876–82.
5. Forman R, Shah S, Jeurissen P, et al. COVID-19 vaccine challenges: What have we learned so far and what remains to be done? Health Policy 2021;125(5): 553–67.
6. Ozdenerol E, Seboly J. The Effects of Lifestyle on COVID-19 Vaccine Hesitancy in the United States: An Analysis of Market Segmentation. Int J Environ Res Public Health 2022;19(13):7732.
7. Mann S, Christini K, Chai Y, et al. Vaccine hesitancy and COVID-19 immunization among rural young adults. Prev Med Rep 2022;28:101845.
8. King WC, Rubinstein M, Reinhart A, et al. Time trends, factors associated with, and reasons for COVID-19 vaccine hesitancy: A massive online survey of US adults from January-May 2021. PLoS One 2021;16(12):e0260731.
9. Kricorian K, Civen R, Equils O. COVID-19 vaccine hesitancy: misinformation and perceptions of vaccine safety. Hum Vaccin Immunother 2022;18(1):1950504.
10. Hasan T, Beardsley J, Marais BJ, et al. The Implementation of Mass-Vaccination against SARS-CoV-2: A Systematic Review of Existing Strategies and Guidelines. Vaccines (Basel) 2021;9(4):326.
11.. Mount Nittany Health. Community Health Needs Assessment. 2019. https://www.mountnittany.org/about-us/community-health-needs-assessment. Accessed 3 June 2022.

12. Evans WD, French J. Demand Creation for COVID-19 Vaccination: Overcoming Vaccine Hesitancy through Social Marketing. Vaccines (Basel) 2021; 9(4):319.
13. Chambers CT, Taddio A, Uman LS, et al, HELPinKIDS Team. Psychological interventions for reducing pain and distress during routine childhood immunizations: a systematic review. Clin Ther 2009;31(Suppl 2):S77–103.

Continuing Nursing Research During a Pandemic

Cynthia K. Snyder, PhD, RN[a], Samantha Acri, MPH[b], Rachel Allen, PhD, PMHNP-BC, RN[c], Mary Louise Kanaskie, PhD, RN, NPD-BC[d],*

KEYWORDS

- COVID-19 • Virtual research • Virtual focus groups • Adolescent sleep research
- Mindfulness research • Code of ethics for nurses • Qualitative research

KEY POINTS

- During the pandemic, established programs of research were able to maintain productivity by being capable of responding swiftly to new guidelines.
- The ability to adapt to new methods and new technology led to research success.
- Virtual platforms created flexible options for study participant enrollment.
- In some studies, virtual formats enabled increased participation and decreased participant attrition.

INTRODUCTION

The coronavirus disease-2019 (COVID-19) pandemic, with its unprecedented infection and fatality rates, disrupted daily life on a magnitude not seen in modern times. Research practices were also disrupted as in-person procedures for nonessential, non-COVID-19 research studies were temporarily suspended by institutions to maximize safety, minimize the spread of infection, and protect individuals' health.[1,2] These disruptions in research practices have drawn attention to the importance of contingency plans to support the continuity of nurse-led clinical research. Events such as the pandemic, which restrict in-person engagement with human subjects require modifications to methods of conducting research.[1–3]

The pandemic also created opportunities to address new research questions.[4] Determining the gaps in our collective knowledge and responding to these needs

Disclosure Statement: The authors (C. Snyder, S. Acri, R. Allen, and M.L. Kanaskie) have no disclosures or funding to report and no commercial or financial conflicts of interest.
a Eastern University, 1300 Eagle Road, Saint Davids, PA 17022, USA; b Systems Analyst Intermediate, Center for Quality Innovation, Penn State Health Shared Services, 90 Hope Drive, Hershey, PA 17033, USA; c College of Nursing, The Pennsylvania State University, 90 Hope Drive, Hershey, PA 17033, USA; d Penn State Health Milton S. Hershey Medical Center, 90 Hope Drive, Hershey, PA 17033, USA
* Corresponding author. 2305 East Tilden Road, Harrisburg, PA 17112.
E-mail address: mlkanaskie@comcast.net

Nurs Clin N Am 58 (2023) 25–34
https://doi.org/10.1016/j.cnur.2022.10.002
0029-6465/23/© 2022 Elsevier Inc. All rights reserved.

required speed in the research process that is seldom seen. Some researchers could build on their earlier work by continuing with the same concepts of interest but adjusting to add new sample populations, adding new ways of delivering an intervention and new methods of data collection. Others responded with new study ideas where timing and relevance became crucial as the pandemic and the accompanying social forces were rapidly changing.

This paper describes several of the challenges that researchers encountered during the COVID-19 pandemic and how the authors have responded. Three research studies are highlighted, which show the following:

1. Using technology to adapt and modify a research proposal
2. Designing a mixed methods study to be totally virtual
3. Conducting virtual focus groups
4. Moving swiftly to retain relevance

In addition, helpful solutions are presented that include various aspects of the research process including subject recruitment, study design, and data collection.

USING TECHNOLOGY TO ADAPT AND MODIFY A RESEARCH STUDY

Readily adapting to changing public health situations requires staying abreast of current local public health guidance and relevant research regulations, as well as competence with available technology. During the pandemic, physical barriers were set that limited person-to-person contacts, administrative barriers to ambulatory care site access, temporary clinic closures, and limitations on numbers of individuals permitted in the clinic.

An original research study, initiated in December 2019 and abruptly halted in March 2020, highlights innovative methods to use technology to move research forward during the COVID-19 pandemic.

Research Case Study 1. Mobile Phones in the Bedroom: Impact on Adolescent Sleep

This descriptive, correlational study sought to explore the attitudes, behaviors, and sleep patterns of adolescents (n = 34; ages 13 to 17) who use mobile phones in the bedroom after lights out. Data were collected via an initial battery of questionnaires on attitudes and beliefs regarding sleep and mobile phone use, followed by a 7-day collection of sleep data via actigraphy (a wristwatch-type device to measure activity as a proxy for sleep), and daily sleep and nighttime mobile phone use diaries. Most of the sample (62%) completed participation before the pause of in-person research, while the remainder were engaged remotely following Institutional Review Board (IRB) approved protocol modifications that allowed for remote engagement.

The study protocol was modified to extend from solely in-person recruitment to also allow remote procedures. This enabled the research to proceed while maintaining compliance with regulatory guidelines. The safe engagement with potential research participants was important to maintain in this study. The study involved two recruitment modalities: in-person recruitment in three ambulatory care sites or via *Studyfinder,* a web-based recruitment database.[5] A detailed description of this web-based study recruitment tool is presented in **Box 1**.

Recruitment was initially slow, with only 10% of the planned recruitment achieved after the first 4 weeks. An unanticipated boost in recruitment occurred after the *Studyfinder* link was posted on personal and local parent group social media pages by a parent.

- Potential study participants or their parents noticed the social media posts and made inquiries about the study through the *Studyfinder* link.

Box 1
Web-Based Recruitment

Web-Based Recruitment.

The use of a web-based recruitment database, such as *Studyfinder*, enables researchers to advertise IRB-approved research studies in a format available for potential participants to: browse available studies, seek additional information from the study team, determine eligibility, and engage in a relevant study.[3,5-7]

Social Media [for example, Facebook, Twitter, and Instagram] can be effective for recruiting: hard to reach populations, large numbers of participants, and people with specific health conditions. In addition, social media may shorten recruitment periods and be cost-effective. The use of social media as a recruitment strategy requires IRB approval with safeguards for participant privacy. Using social media may exclude those without internet or broadband access resulting in bias and limiting generalizability of findings.[3,6]

- This occurrence resulted in snowball recruitment as parents or their adolescents shared the information among peer networks, providing greater exposure within the local community with enhanced interest in study participation.
- Snowball recruitment may result in selection bias limiting generalizability of results. More than half of the study participants were recruited before the cessation of in-person clinical research activities.
- Study recruitment continued via *Studyfinder* only, which enabled participant recruitment to be completed within the original timeline. Initially, the study protocol involved in-person enrollment with signed parental consent and minor assent at the initial study visit.
- After suspension of in-person research activities, remote enrollment via secure Zoom videoconference was implemented following consultation with an Office of Research Protection analyst, subsequent study modification, and IRB approval.

Remote enrollment included evaluation of screening questions, explanation of the study with participant expectations, and verbal consent and minor assent, which was followed by return of a signed consent via email (**Box 2**). This successful strategy also facilitated flexible enrollment on evenings and weekends when participants and parents were less likely to be occupied.

Electronic data capture (EDC) with *Research Electronic Data Capture* (REDCap) was planned and conducted from the outset of the study and continued during the suspension of in-person research. Remote options for data collection are described in **Box 3**.

- REDCap enabled direct data entry by participants with twice daily e-mail prompts and eliminated handling of paper forms and manual entry of data.
- The wrist actigraphy watch device was issued at study enrollment and participants began the 7-day data collection immediately. However, following the transition to remote enrollment, this device was mailed to participants via the postal service and data collection began upon receipt of the device.
- Distribution of research study devices that are needed to collect data is traditionally done in person; however, alternate methods of device distribution are required during a pandemic. Alternatives include the use of the postal service, shipping companies, or private couriers to transport data collection devices.

> **Box 2**
> **Study Screening and Enrollment**
>
> Web-based screening and enrollment tools.
>
> Web-based screening tools, such as Survey Monkey or Qualtrix, as well as electronic data systems such as *Research Electronic Data Capture* (REDCap) are resources which may be used to screen potential participants safely.[2,3] Parental consent and minor assent may occur electronically or verbally (eg, telephone; videoconference).
>
> Secure videoconferences via BlueJeans for Health care, Go To Meeting, Microsoft Teams, or Zoom for Health care facilitate remote approaches for consent/assent (Stiles-Shields et al., 2020).[2] Electronic resources (eg, DocuSign; REDCap; Qualtrix) enable electronic signatures indicating consent and minor assent.[2,3]

Traditional participant incentives frequently take the forms of physical gift cards, checks, or cash payments. An adaptation is electronic gift cards or reloadable debit cards. Each can be easily purchased and sent directly to participants via email.[2,3]

DESIGNING A STUDY TO BE TOTALLY VIRTUAL

Research Case Study 2. Nurses evaluate whether a mindfulness intervention decreases stress (NEW MINDS)

Planning for the NEW MINDS (Nurses Evaluate Whether a Mindfulness Intervention Nets Decreased Stress) study began in 2019 with brainstorming sessions including members of the Research and Evidence-based Practice Council. The study team, including three clinical nurses, an advanced practice nurse, a nursing faculty member, and a statistician, collaborated with a clinical psychologist, who is a certified mindfulness-based stress reduction (MBSR) instructor.[11] The team decided to focus on two major sets of stress-related outcomes to measure the impact of mindfulness training for bedside nurses—physiologic measurements and self-reported measurements (surveys and focus groups).

Two intervention groups were designed for comparison: a full MBSR course and an abbreviated mindfulness training program. All study activities including obtaining informed consent, study orientation, MBSR training sessions, and data collection sessions (surveys, focus groups, and physiologic measurements) were designed to be conducted in-person during defined meeting times.

By June 2020, the team had received sufficient funding to support the cost of the mindfulness training program materials and instructor, and developed an agreement to collect all physiologic measurements using one of the study team member's labs at no additional cost to the study team. All study protocol and supporting documents were written in preparation for submission to the IRB.

Shortly thereafter, conditions began to change regarding community transmission of COVID-19 and resulting hospitalizations. In response to local and federal restrictions, the University guidance, and other factors, research laboratory occupancy was reduced to 25% of normal operating occupancy, and funding was severely reduced. As a result, the study team received notification in late July 2020 that all outcomes based on physiologic measurements would have to be removed from the study protocol. The laboratory resources were simply not available to carry out that aspect of the study. Despite these challenges, the team decided that the importance of the mindfulness interventions (especially in the context of a pandemic) and the potential knowledge gained from self-reported measurements made it possible to simply exclude the physiologic measurements and move forward with the remainder of the study.

> **Box 3**
> **Data Collection: Remote Options**
>
> Remote Options for Data Collection.
>
> Remote options for data collection include Electronic Data Capture (EDC) (eg, REDCap, ConnEDCt, Qualtrix, Survey Monkey, Excel), phone, telehealth, home-based monitoring, or videoconference modalities.[1,2,8,9]
>
> The use of an EDC platform requires orientation, training, and testing before IRB approval. The REDCap system enables researchers to collect, store, and export data to statistical software packages for analysis.[8] The ConnEDCt data base system was developed to collect and manage public health data,[8] whereas the Comprehensive Adolescent Research and Engagement Studies (CARES) EDC was developed specifically for management of HIV data.[10]

The team quickly adjusted the protocol and supporting documents, and in September 2020, the study was approved by the IRB. Dates and locations for the mindfulness training courses were determined and planning for recruitment began. As the study was preparing to launch, though, the notification came from the Office of Human Protections that all in-person study activities were being suspended. This meant that all in-person meetings for the study (consent, orientation, data collection, MBSR course) would have to be delayed until after the restrictions were lifted or that we would have to convert to a totally virtual study—unfamiliar territory for the majority of the study team. Considering the unknown timeline of COVID-19 and the safety of our study team and participants, conversion to a virtual format was chosen. By mid-October, a modified version of the study was resubmitted and approved by the IRB. The study timeline with redesign steps is shown in **Fig. 1**.

The revisions included a redesign for three major aspects of the study:

1. The process to obtain and document informed consent from each participant was now conducted entirely virtually, rather than in-person.
   - A study team member set up a meeting with each interested nurse after an email exchange to check eligibility and determine the participant's intervention group of choice (interventions were not randomly allocated due to the significant differences in scheduling commitment).

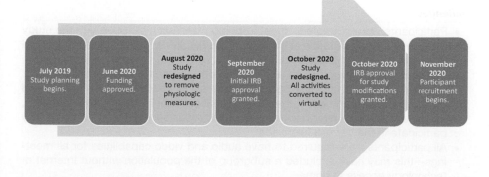

Fig. 1. New MINDS study timeline.

- Using an online survey form developed in close collaboration with the IRB, the study team member reviewed the whole consent form with the participant and answered questions and then both parties signed and dated the form.
2. Orientation and MBSR course sessions were now held virtually.
   - Mindfulness training courses are traditionally held in-person to enhance the shared experience of connectedness and support among participants.
   - The team originally intended for one group to enroll in a traditional MBSR program (in-person class held 2 to 3 h weekly for 8 weeks plus a day-long silent retreat), whereas the other group received an abbreviated, pre-recorded version of the course material meant to only take a few minutes each week after an initial in-person training session.
   - With the study redesign, both groups' interventions were now fully virtual.
3. All surveys were now sent electronically.
   - Participants complete the surveys at their own convenience (within an allotted time frame) rather than asking all participants to attend in-person data collection sessions with printed survey forms.
   - Focus groups were also conducted virtually.

By transforming to a fully virtual study, we found a variety of benefits and challenges which will help to inform future studies.

Benefits

- Virtual training made accessibility much easier—no one had to worry about driving to attend the course at a physical location, and participants could join from practically anywhere as long as connection was available. For example, one participant in the full MBSR group drove to the beach to get the most relaxing experience for the full-day silent retreat.
- The study team and the participant had immediate access to the signed consent document by using the virtual consent process, and there was no need for secure storage protocols for paper-based consent forms.
- Data collection via electronic surveys allowed participants to enter and submit their responses privately without any involvement of the study team (other than sending survey invitations and reminders). This removed the possibility of data entry mistakes. Also, no need for storing paper forms again.
- Conducting virtual focus groups may have allowed participants to speak more freely and honestly than they would have in-person.

Challenges

- Participants were not able to meet in-person with each other or with the study team for the whole duration of the study. This resulted in some frustration related to the lack of personal connection.
- Materials such as yoga mats and meditation cushions are generally provided during in-person mindfulness training programs. Because there was no physical contact with any participant, these materials could not be distributed; therefore, participants may or may not have had the proper equipment at home to fully participate in the training exercises.
- All participants were required to have audio and video capabilities for all meetings—this may have excluded a subgroup of the population without Internet or technology access at home.
- Although it has its advantages, allowing participants to join virtually from anywhere for all study activities made eliminating distractions a challenge. Each

participant was in the setting of their choice rather than a controlled, consistent environment. It is possible that participants in a chaotic environment (at work, with children and/or pets in the background, etc.) may have struggled to focus and learn from the mindfulness interventions to the same degree as participants in a secluded/quiet learning environment.

- In-person MBSR courses are the "gold standard" intervention when it comes to mindfulness training.[11] Because all study activities were converted to virtual meetings, neither of our intervention groups met the traditional course standards.

With the study changes made and approved, recruitment eventually launched in November 2020 and the interventions began in January 2021.

In addition to the challenges surrounding the conversion to a virtual study, the difficult personal and work-related situations caused by the COVID-19 pandemic led to some study recruitment and retention challenges as well. Out of the 45 participants that we intended to enroll in the "brief" mindfulness training course, 39 nurses (in two waves of 29 then 10) joined the study and 25 of them completed the intervention and participated in pre- and post-intervention data collection. For the full MBSR course group, 14 nurses were enrolled out of the 15 available spots, and 10 of them completed the intervention and data collection. Increased time commitment, changing schedules, and staffing challenges at work during surges of COVID-19 hospitalization as well as personal/family conflicts explained the majority of study non-completion.

CONDUCTING VIRTUAL FOCUS GROUPS

The qualitative data for the NEW MINDS mixed methods study was collected in semi-structured focus group interviews lasting approximately 1 h, conducted 3 months post-intervention, and repeated at 9 months post-intervention. Initial focus groups and follow-up focus groups were facilitated by two consistent nurse researchers. Focus groups were conducted via a virtual platform as necessitated by the COVID-19 pandemic. This format presented potential challenges to the facilitators, as well as unexpected benefits.

Benefits

Virtual focus groups offered a significant advantage to participants, and consequently, the overall quality of the study. Based on feedback from participants:

1. The virtual format allowed for easier participation in the focus groups, as participants only needed to accommodate a designated time, and not a designated location. Some participants lived an hour or more away from the hospital that served as the study location, and reported that they would not have been inclined to travel back to the hospital for the focus groups.
2. Conducting focus groups virtually eliminated the need for facilitators to reserve appropriate meeting space for the focus group in advance, and avoid potential space scheduling conflicts.
3. Participant feedback supported the conclusion that rather than functioning as a barrier, the virtual format instead enabled increased participation in the focus groups, and decreased participant attrition.

Similarly, the increased flexibility and convenience afforded by the virtual platform to participants also enabled the focus group facilitators to offer a greater variety of time/day options for focus groups without considerations for travel time, child care, or other constraints. The range of times and days increased access for participants by accommodating their individual work shifts and personal schedules. Participants who were isolating or on quarantine were still able to participate and attend virtually as well.

Finally, a benefit to the virtual format of the study was the integrated recording feature of the virtual platform. The integrated recording capability streamlined the focus group recording process, necessary for transcription and qualitative analysis while ensuring that each participant's active consent was recorded.

Barriers

Despite the overwhelmingly positive experience with the virtual platform for the focus groups, this format posed several potential barriers in executing focus groups. By anticipating these challenges and adapting accordingly, the facilitators were able to overcome them.

1. One such concern was the ability to ensure the anonymity of focus group participants in the virtual format. This was addressed by the facilitators disabling the Zoom platform's display of participants' names in their respective video windows.
2. The virtual format presented a possible barrier to study participants with decreased comfort/familiarity with technology, and opened up the potential for technological difficulties. In preparation for this possibility, one of the focus group facilitators was designated to assist with technological difficulties if needed, whereas the other facilitator conducted the interview. Fortunately, these problems did not materialize, as all facilitators and participants had prior experience using the virtual platform.
3. Facilitators were tasked with creating a comfortable, welcoming focus group environment over a virtual platform while establishing rapport with and among participants.

Benefits and challenges to using virtual methods for conducting qualitative research have been reported by other researchers who have made similar observations.[12,13] Ultimately, in this study, focus group facilitators determined that they were able to create an appropriate atmosphere for active participation and honest feedback from participants in the focus group despite the virtual format.

Unexpected Findings

The greatest unexpected finding to arise from the pandemic-imposed process of conducting focus groups virtually was that facilitators were still able to cultivate meaningful connections with and among participants and foster a safe and open space for discussion through virtual means. The significance of this finding, while not conclusive, cannot be overlooked, especially regarding its potential bearing upon other studies that may require qualitative data collection and analysis to be conducted virtually.

MOVING SWIFTLY TO RETAIN RELEVANCE

Adaptability during the pandemic was essential for research productivity. This was true for bench researchers who had the vision to adapt their labs and equipment to contribute in new ways to address the public health crisis; as well as for researchers in the social sciences and nursing. Researchers moved swiftly to meet immediate life-saving needs, as well as to study the human experience in real time.

The COVID-19 pandemic has challenged nurses and all health care professionals to examine how we balance the obligation to provide safe care to those in need while also meeting obligations to self-care. In addition, long-standing infection control practices were altered as we struggled to find and maintain adequate supplies of personal protective equipment (PPE). As the months progressed, supplies became available but another valuable resource challenge emerged. In the fall of 2021, the shortage of registered nurses to provide care to the sick and to the well in all practice settings was a problem without a solution in site.

The ANA Code of Ethics for Nurses has a long tradition of providing moral guidance for all nurses in all practice domains.[14] "The Code is one standard that is universally applicable to all nurses."[15] For these reasons, it provided an excellent framework to study how nurses were practicing, coping, and the resources they needed to continue.

Research Case Study 3. Ethics in an era of the pandemic.

Nurse researchers at our institution set out to understand the experience of nurses during the first stage of COVID-19 by studying the relevance of the ANA Code of Ethics to their practice during the pandemic.[16]

A descriptive study using qualitative methods was conducted with nurses participating in one of six virtual focus groups. Twenty-three registered nurses participated. They represented acute care and ambulatory care settings; cared for adults, children and families; cared for patients with COVID-19 infections, many of who were critically ill. The ANA Code of Ethics was shared and participants were asked to identify which provisions, if any, seemed most relevant to their practice during COVID-19. Findings indicated that most of the provisions had relevance. There was a strong appreciation for collaborative efforts and a strong sense of obligation and commitment. Nurses served as advocates for patients, families, and communities. They witnessed increased suffering and death and identified the need for palliative care education and struggled to maintain a work–life balance.[16]

In studying the experience of a pandemic as it is occurring, research processes and timelines needed to move faster than usual for findings to maintain their relevance. In this study, nurse researchers were able to move swiftly by using their knowledge and expertise in bioethics and qualitative research methods to design and implement the study within 3 months. In addition, moving quickly on research dissemination through publications and presentations became equally important. Writing of the initial manuscript began while data analysis was underway and attention to abstract submission deadlines to national conferences was paramount.

SUMMARY

The COVID-19 pandemic altered traditional methods of conducting clinical research and required nurse researchers to adapt research protocols to the new guidelines. In-person research was largely replaced by remote processes with integration of electronic resources into all aspects of research approaches. Researcher preparedness, flexibility, and perseverance were strengths that promoted research success. In addition, prompt assessment of barriers and facilitators to continued research amid an uncertain environment was critically important.

Researchers conducting clinical research during a pandemic can benefit from: acknowledging the challenges faced; staying virtually connected with one another, participants, study sites, and advisory board members; and regular brainstorming to benefit from the team's combined ingenuity, resources, skills, and networks. Taken together, these approaches can maintain study integrity, while promoting recruitment, enrollment, and engagement with research participants, so that data may be collected and analyzed and findings may be disseminated within (or close to) the study timeline.

The question looms as to the long-term impact of remote research practices and if modifications adopted during the COVID-19 pandemic will become standard operating procedures. This recent public health crisis should serve as a call to action for research teams to evaluate current processes and procedures, team members' skill sets and knowledge of current and emerging technological advancements. Although technology offers innovative methods in meeting current research needs, it is not without challenges and continued need for ethics evaluation.

CLINICS CARE POINTS

- Embracing the use of technology in clinical research can potentially help with all stages of a study: subject recruitment and enrollment, providing interventions, and delivering incentives.

- Virtual platforms may provide focus group facilitators the ability to make connections with and among participants and foster a safe and open space for discussion.

- In studying the experience of a pandemic as it is occurring, research processes and timelines need to move faster than usual for findings to maintain their relevance.

REFERENCES

1. Omary MB, Eswaraka J, Kimball SD, et al. The COVID-19 pandemic and research shutdown: Staying safe and productive. JCI 2020;130(6):1–8.
2. Stiles-Shields B, Plevinsky JM, Psihogios AM, et al. Considerations and future directions for conducting clinical research with pediatric populations during the COVID-19 pandemic. JPP 2020;45:720–4.
3. Saberi P. Research in the time or coronavirus: Continuing ongoing studies in the midst of the COVID-19 pandemic. AIDS Behav 2020;24(8):2232–5.
4. Speroni KG, Hess R. Pandemic challenges: Keeping nursing research alive. JONA 2021;51(7/8):364–5.
5. Studyfinder 2022. Available at. https://studyfinder.psu.edu/researchers. Accessed date June 21, 2022.
6. Topolovec-Vranic J, Natarajan K. The use of social media in recruitment for medical research studies: A scoping review. J Med Internet Res 2016;18(11):e286.
7. Gelinas L, Pierce R, Winkler S, et al. Using social media as a research recruitment tool: Ethical issues and recommendations. Am J Bioeth 2017;17:3–14.
8. Harris PA, Taylor R, Thielke R, et al. Research Electronic Data Capture (REDCap)—A metadata-driven methodology and workflow process for providing translational research informatics support. J Biomed Inform 2009;42:377–81.
9. Ruth CJ, Huey SL, Krisher JT, et al. An electronic data capture framework (ConnEDCt) for global and public health research: Design and implementation. J Med Internet Res 2020;22(8):e18580.
10. Comulada WS, Tang W, Swendeman D, et al. Development of an electronic data collection system to support a large-scale HIV behavioral intervention trial: protocol for an electronic data collection system. JMIR Res Protoc 2018;7(12):e10777.
11. Leader Mindful. What is Mindfulness-Based Stress Reduction (MBSR)?. Available at: https://www.mindfulleader.org/. Accessed June 23, 2022.
12. Schlegel EC, Tate JA. Pickler RH, Smith, LH. Practical strategies for qualitative inquiry in a virtual world. J Adv Nurs 2021;77(10):4035–44.
13. Pocock T, Smith M, Wiles J. Recommendations for Virtual Qualitative Health Research During a Pandemic. Qual Health Res 2021;31(13):2403–13.
14. American Nurses Association. Code of ethics for nurses with Interpretative Statements. Silver Spring (MD): American Nurses Association; 2015.
15. Fowler MD. Faith and Ethics, Covenant and Code. J Christ Nurs 2017;34(4):216–24.
16. Dellasega C. Kanaskie ML Nursing ethics in an era of pandemic. Appl Nurs Res 2021;62:151508.

Long-Term Care and the COVID-19 Pandemic

Lessons Learned

Marie Boltz, PhD, GNP-BC

KEYWORDS

- Long-term care • Nurses • COVID-19 strategies • Nursing home • Assisted living
- Adult day services

KEY POINTS

- Approximately 74% of the deaths in the US COVID-19 have occurred in adults aged 65 years and older due to intrinsic vulnerabilities including comorbidity and frailty and residence in communal living spaces.
- Across all long-term care settings older adults were challenged by both the threat of COVID-19 infection as well as the unintended consequences of restricted visitation and isolation practices including loneliness, depression, delirium, functional decline, and nutritional problems.
- A trauma-informed approach is necessary to address the stresses and losses of older adults, family, and staff.

INTRODUCTION

Approximately 74% of the deaths in the United States from severe acute respiratory syndrome coronavirus 2 (SARS-CoV-2) that causes COVID-19 have occurred in adults age 65 years and older.[1] Intrinsic vulnerabilities include comorbidity and frailty; residence in communal living spaces considered "hot spots" have contributed to higher risk.[2] US nursing homes (NHs) and other long-term care (LTC) communities such as assisted living and adult day care services have been disproportionally affected by COVID-19.[2–6] Nurses and health care workers provided care and services despite health concerns for themselves and family members. Nurses on the frontline were called to act with extraordinary tenacity, skill, flexibility, and creativity.[7] The purpose of this article is to provide an overview of the challenges posed by the COVID-19 pandemic in LTC settings and the strategies prioritized and implemented with interdisciplinary colleagues in NHs, assisted living, and adult day services.

Ross and Carol Nese College of Nursing, Penn State, 302 Nursing Sciences Building, University Park, PA 16802, USA
E-mail address: mpb40@psu.edu
Twitter: @MarieBoltz1 (M.B.)

Nurs Clin N Am 58 (2023) 35–48
https://doi.org/10.1016/j.cnur.2022.10.004
0029-6465/23/© 2022 Elsevier Inc. All rights reserved.

THE NURSING HOME CONTEXT, STRATEGIES, AND LESSONS LEARNED

The most severely affected by COVID-19 were residents in the approximately 15,400 NHs, also referred to as skilled nursing facilities.[2,3,8,9] Individual states have reported that up to 50% of cases and deaths attributed to the virus have occurred in these facilities.[4] These care communities are certified by Medicare and/or Medicaid and include almost 1.3 million residents in the United States.[5] Most NHs provide both LTC for residents with high care dependency and complex health care needs, as well as short-term, postacute care for patients admitted from the hospital who require highly skilled nursing care and/or rehabilitation.[9] Short-term posthospital care is largely reimbursed by Medicaid, whereas most LTC is reimbursed by Medicaid.[9,10] NHs that are predominantly dependent on Medicaid have less resources and lower staffing levels, are located in the poorest neighborhoods, and have the most quality problems.[10] Nursing home residents have many of the comorbidities that are considered risk factors for COVID-19 mortality (cardiovascular diseases, diabetes, chronic respiratory disorders, hypertension, and cancer).[9]

Research on the facility characteristics associated with higher COVID-19 cases are conflicting. Some research indicated that NHs with low RN and total staffing levels have seemed to leave residents vulnerable to COVID-19 infections.[11,12] Lower nursing home quality ratings (overall quality rating of 1 to 5 stars based on performance on 3 domains, each rated on 1 to 5 stars: health inspections, nurse staffing, and resident quality measures) were also found to be associated with higher COVID-19 incidence, mortality, and persistence.[12–14] In contrast, it was the location of a nursing home, asymptomatic spread, and availability of testing—not quality ratings, infection citations or staffing—that were found to be determining factors in COVID-19 outbreaks, according to independent analyses by leading academic and health care experts, as well as government researchers.[15–18] Larger facility size, urban location, and a greater percentage of African American residents were also associated with higher rates of infection.[15] A study of 12,576 US NHs, conducted by Li and colleagues[12] found that NHs with higher numbers of racial and ethnic minorities reported greater incidences of confirmed COVID-19 cases and deaths. In addition, in a cohort study of US nursing home residents with COVID-19, increased age, male sex, and impaired cognitive and physical function were independently associated with mortality.[19]

Nurse Leaders Influencing Policy

NHs experienced a steep learning curve during the COVID-19 pandemic.[20–23] NHs were required to quickly mobilize to implement the use of personal protective equipment (PPE), testing, and restrictive visitation policies. The fast spread of COVID-19 challenged federal and state agencies to provide timely guidance and NHs to implement those changes and still meet the daily health care needs of their residents.[3] Nurse leaders assumed a critical role at the national and facility level to provide information, develop and help implement policy, and educate staff. For example, Deb Bakerjian developed and continues to update the Web site, "Coronavirus Disease 2019 (COVID-19) and Safety of Older Adults Residing in Nursing Homes" on the Agency for Healthcare Research and Quality (AHRQ) Patient Safety network. The primer is a compilation of information that has affected the safety of older adults and has been published on federal Web sites, in professional and academic literature and in the press.[3]

A critical nursing role that has been highlighted by the pandemic is the infection preventionist (IP). The Centers for Medicare and Medicaid Services (CMS) in October 2016 expanded NH infection prevention and control (IPC) requirements to include an antibiotic stewardship program and a designated individual to serve as an IP to oversee the program[24]; this was based on research demonstrating that NHs with IPs who had specialized training were 5 to 13 times more likely to have a stronger IPC program.[24] Before pandemic, IPs typically had multiple roles and thus are not able to dedicate their full time to IPC.[25] The pandemic illuminated the need for a full-time essential IP to coordinate interdisciplinary activity including tracking cases of infection, educating staff, overseeing testing, and monitoring facility IPC practices.[26,27]

The California state nursing workforce center (HealthImpact) partnered with nurse leaders within the state to address macrolevel nursing workforce issues during the pandemic. Academic and clinical practice nurse leaders created guidance documents for schools of nursing and clinical agencies to support and encourage safe academic-practice partnerships during the pandemic.[28] The coalition worked with the California Board of Registered Nursing to also create official guidance documents to explain the various roles nursing students can assume to contribute to the workforce during the pandemic. They developed free high-quality simulations and supported a bill that codified the governor's waiver for increased use of simulation in disaster situations. The coalition also created a toolkit to help introduce or refresh essential knowledge for retired nurse returning to the workforce and nursing students and worked with other nurse leader organizations to create resources, webinars, and podcasts to support the well-being and health of nurses. Finally, the coalition created a volunteer registration and matching system for interprofessional health care licensees and students to staff vaccination events throughout California especially in communities of color and hard-to-reach communities.[28]

The CMS recognized the urgency of the COVID-19 crisis and convened the Coronavirus Commission for Safety and Quality in NHs in April, 2020.[29] The 25-member commission was composed of academicians, clinicians, NH administrators, family members, residents, industry professionals, and scientific experts. The members were charged with making recommendations to improve infection prevention and control, safety procedures, and the quality of life of residents in NHs. The final report of the Commission contained 27 recommendations and was released in September 2020.[29] A group of geriatric nurse experts responded to this report and while confirming the committee's observations, posited that there were other policy weaknesses that have been long-standing problems and exacerbated the COVID-19 crisis. The experts identified weaknesses including chronic overall understaffing and insufficient numbers of professional nurses (that is, registered nurses [RNs]), insufficient geriatric expertise for managing complex care problems, and a culture focused on regulatory compliance, to the exclusion of quality improvement.[21] Consequently, the nurse experts made the following recommendations: (1) ensuring RN coverage on a daily, around the clock basis and providing adequate compensation to provide total staffing levels that are commensurate with the needs of the residents; (2) ensuring RNs have both clinical and leadership competencies in geriatric nursing, including quality improvement and supervisory skills; (3) increasing efforts to recruit and retain the NH workforce, particularly RNs; and (4) supporting care delivery models, including the professional practice model, that strengthen the role of the RN.[22,23,30]

Care of Residents and Families

In addition to enormous mortality and morbidity, nursing home residents faced the unintended consequences of restricted visitation and isolation practices that were implemented to curtail exposure to COVID-19.[31–37] NHs reported that that residents had stopped eating and had "given up" without family visitation.[38] Residents were confined to their rooms, precluding their engagement in communal meals, activities, and normal levels of physical activity, all factors associated with delirium, nutritional problems, psychological distress, functional decline, and falls.[38–40] A scoping review of restricted visitation described significant mental health consequences for the patient, including anxiety, loneliness, depressive symptoms, agitation, aggression, reduced cognitive ability, and overall dissatisfaction.[41] Residents' families were also negatively affected by this practice; lack of connectivity with loved ones added an additional layer of stress to the worry and anxiety they experienced in the face of the pandemic crisis.[40]

Simple interventions promoted connectivity with families. For example, families were encouraged to drop off letters, drawings, or other packages and maintain contact with regular telephone check-ins.[41] Video calls for residents to interact virtually with their families have been shown to decrease depressive symptoms, loneliness, and increase social interaction and quality of life.[42–45] However, many NHs do not have the resources to promote everyday technology use to enable residents to connect with providers and families, which worsened health disparities.[45–47] For example, a study conducted by Savage and colleagues[47] found that residents who did not have personal contact, including phone calls, with loved ones during COVID-19 restrictions experienced 35% greater excess mortality compared with residents who had personal contact. When tablets and laptops have been made available, nursing staff have reported benefits such as increased resident well-being and increased family engagement in care plan meetings.[36,47,48] In addition, staff described greater ease in educating families and connecting the residents to health care consultants.[48,49] Resident unfamiliarity with technology and staff concern about technology being an additional burden have been barriers. However, studies demonstrated that residents were receptive to technology and technology actually reduced staff burden by keeping residents engaged and freeing up staff for other activities.[43,44] Another technology known as simulated presence therapy, whereby recorded video messages from family or friends are replayed frequently, led to the enhanced well-being of residents living with dementia and decreased behavioral symptoms of distress.[37]

The pandemic also demanded excellent basic nursing care.[41] Nursing staff have reported that the use of face masks that have a clear window has helped with communication with residents. Preference congruence and positive interactions were supported by interdisciplinary assessment of the residents' psychosocial needs, backgrounds, and preferences.[41,49,50] Improvement initiatives focused on measures such as structured, consistent rounding to provide cognitive stimulation and social interaction, snacks and fluids, physical activity. The use of exergames have been shown to improve functional capacity and increased interaction with other residents, families, and friends. In addition, simple approaches to increase physical activity, including sit-to-stand exercises, walking, and encouragement of self-care in hygiene and grooming, could be incorporated into rounds and room visitations.[51–54]

Trauma-Informed Care

For residents, staff, and families, the COVID-19 pandemic has been marked by isolation, uncertainty, and loss, all hallmarks of trauma.[55] The Substance Abuse and Mental Health Services Administration (SAMHSA) guidelines define trauma as an event or pattern of occurrences that is experienced as harmful or threatening and has ongoing negative effects on the person.[56] Viewing the pandemic as traumatic underscores the need to provide support to mitigate the effects of trauma. LTC residents' response to trauma can present as increased anxiety, agitation, aggression, or withdrawal. Cornerstones of trauma-informed care include trying to understand the person (knowing the person, looking for the reason behind behavior), acting with empathy, engaging the person's social support, and providing choice whenever possible. The mainstay of treatment is nonpharmacological interventions including communicating and acting with empathy.[57] Trauma experts have provided guidance during the pandemic to support the well-being of all members of the NH community, in the face of trauma that feels unrelenting and tests resilience. **Box 1** provides a summary for increasing compassion resiliency and moral wellness.[58]

Nursing home staff were particularly exposed and vulnerable to COVID-19. Many of these workers struggle with grief over the suffering they have witnessed, both at work and in their communities. Some have been infected with COVID-19 and recovered physically—but not emotionally. In addition to many experiencing COVID illness, staff at all levels described dramatic levels of personal distress, including feelings of helplessness, fear, and anxiety.[58] Balancing high, often concurrent, and competing demands of work and family was reported as a major source of stress. There was frustration with operational challenges including inadequate access to personal protective equipment and COVID testing and lack of information and consistent guidance.[59] Moreover, staff were dealing with their grief when residents died.

Attention to signs of burnout, difficulty coping, and substance misuse have required promote attention and referral to employee assistance programs and mental health professionals.

Strategies that NHs have implemented to support staff well-being include attention to the work environment including ensuring sufficient supply of PPE; consistency in assigned units; and clear, direct, and frequent communication from supervisors. Another strategy included instituting formal, scripted pauses at set times or debriefing after resident deaths or other stressful events. Moments of pause and huddles to acknowledge and verbalize difficulties and promote safe discussion have been helpful. Nurse administrators have also promoted staff morale and well-being through numerous small acts such as acknowledging team members for their work contributions, celebrating patient recoveries, and highlighting recognition from patients and families.[60,61]

The pandemic crisis has demanded administrators and managers that are consistently present; attentive to multiple sources of information; nimble in their planning and responses; and effective in their communication with staff, residents, and families.

Box 1
Supporting compassion resiliency and moral wellness in postacute and long-term care settings: best practices

- Refrain From Offering Nonempathic Responses
  - Avoid giving advice, telling your own story, and interrogating

- Offer Empathic Responses
  - Use empathic *reflection* (It sounds like......Am I right?)

- Pause When Starting to Get Reactive and Choose Your Response
  - Be aware of your physical and emotional reaction

- Decrease Blame
  - Consider the other person's experience
  - Try to figure out what matters most to the person

- Create Empathic Support Structures
  - Agree on how you can support the other person (eg, checking on at certain times of day).

Adapted from Beausoleil.[58]

Practical operational tools are essential to support these practices. A large, urban LTC facility, Louis Brier Home and Hospital, developed a comprehensive check-list for easy review of measurable indicators associated with 12 infection control practices and policies. A list of the policies and practices developed by Havaei and colleagues[50] are shared in **Box 2**. The nurse leaders complement these items with measurable indicators.

The Role of the Nurse Practitioner in COVID-19–Related Care

Nurse practitioners have a proven track record of providing safe and cost-effective care in LTC, improving resident outcomes, in the areas of polypharmacy, falls, restraint use, and transfers to acute care and thus are well positioned to lead and respond to the complexity of COVID-19 care.[62–65] In addition to conducting comprehensive assessments, rapid recognition and response to clinical deterioration, symptomatic care, psychological support, and prevention of multiple potential complications, nurse practitioners provided other critical functions. Qualitative research with nurse practitioners described the foci of their work during the pandemic. They described the responsibilities associated with containing the spread of COVID-19 within the LTC homes, including working with management to implement and communicate the evolving COVID-19 recommendations from local health authorities and implement pandemic protocols such as resident cohorting and isolation plans, testing, and infection control practices. In many cases, the nurse practitioners provided the in-person clinical visits with residents when the physicians were making virtual visits only. A third critical function was providing emotional support to fearful staff and residents' families and education about the pandemic and resident care needs. Maintaining relationships between residents and their families was also a focus of the clinicians' work. Finally, the nurse practitioners acted as a liaison with other health care systems including acute care, home care, and emergency departments and worked with them to create policies, strategies, and algorithms to minimize fragmentation in care.[66]

Box 2
Items in the check-list of best practice policies for nursing leaders

- Screening
- Visitor policies
- Hand hygiene
- Respiratory hygiene and PPE
- Source control and physical distancing
- Point-of-care risk assessment
- Cleaning and disinfecting
- Suspected and confirmed COVID-19 cases
- Psychological support for residents
- Psychological support for staff
- Monitoring (eg, staff levels, PPE availability)
- Communication (eg, COVID-19 emergency response team, accessible response plan)

Adapted from Havaei, MacPhee, Keselman and Staempfli.[50]

In another study nurse practitioners described the complexity of their roles in promoting a dignified death for LTC residents during the COVID-19 pandemic.[67] They described intensive engagement with residents and more frequently their care partners, to facilitate advance care planning and goals of care conversations. The nurse practitioners promoted comfort at end of life by prescribing pharmacologic and non-pharmacologic interventions symptom management; consulting with expert clinicians where needed; addressing the psychosocial needs of residents and families, and providing education to staff on comfort measures. Nurse practitioners also facilitated compassionate visits to care partners when their residents were imminently dying, allowing them to stay as long as possible while making sure that their PPE remained safely useable. The nurse practitioners also described "care after death," which included informing the care partners of the death, upholding the pandemic-related policy of allowing only one grieving care partner at a time, and completing death certificates. They also educated and often supervised safe care of the resident's body after death. A good deal of time was spent providing emotional support to staff, with minimal time to focus on in their own self-care.[67]

Experts in advanced practice registered nurse (APRN) practice have recommended that APRNs (both nurse practitioners and clinical specialists) use their leadership skills to provide consultation and lead quality improvement efforts beyond the COVID-19 pandemic. There is a critical need to use evidence of past successes to influence NH owners, operators, and policy makers to extend and strengthen the APRN role in LTC.[68,69]

ASSISTED LIVING AND ADULT DAY SERVICE: CONTEXT, STRATEGIES, AND LESSONS LEARNED
Assisted Living

More than 800,000 residents live in the 28,000 US assisted living facilities (ALFs); 52% are age 85 years and older and 30% are between the ages of 75 and 84 years. ALFs are not licensed as health care facilities; they do not provide round-the-clock skilled nursing care. There are no federal regulations for ALFs, and state regulations vary considerably. ALFs also vary widely in the array of services provided, ranging from around the clock assistance with daily living to on-call assistance. ALF care is largely private pay, although a small amount is reimbursed via Medicaid waiver programs. Some ALFs specialize in the care of people with dementia and other forms of cognitive impairment.[70]

The staffing, structure, and resources of ALFs limit the capacity of ALFs to respond to the COVID-19 outbreak.[71] The staff are largely unlicensed direct care workers, and the number of nurses varies widely. Unlike NHs, there is no requirement for a medical director or an infection control practitioner. There are also no standard requirements for infection control or an infection control practitioner, as there are in NHs. Residents may receive care from their personal medical provider; they are not required to have regular medical visits. Residents often rely on external providers to provide home care attendants in their own apartment or rooms. Although residents could be restricted to their rooms, it would require significant staff to provide needed care and residents would need to agree to adhere to such restrictions, which makes it difficult to enforce such universal precautions. This structure is also not as conducive as NHs to cohort residents. Consequently, ALFs have relied on close collaboration with local health authorities and service agencies to guide infection control practices and monitoring.[71–73]

Approximately 42% of assisted living residents have dementia, who may be particularly vulnerable to the adverse effects of social isolation and loneliness from visitor restriction and curtailing of group activities.[37,40] The overall lower numbers of staff and lack of a requirement for a nurse on staff predispose the residents to complications including falls, dehydration/nutritional problems, and delirium. Advanced practice RNs and home care nurses with palliative care expertise have been engaged in some ALFs and in some instances have addressed these challenges. In one ALF, in Washington, the palliative care nurse collaborated with APRNs to triage residents, manage symptoms, coordinate the functions of the interdisciplinary team, and monitor health patterns among all residents. A dedicated palliative RN was enlisted to coordinate prompt goals of care conversations with all residents, which was necessary because of the rapid deterioration of some residents once they became symptomatic. The palliative team supplemented the efforts of the remaining staff to provide an extra layer of support to meet the social, emotional, and spiritual needs of the residents who were finding themselves suddenly shut off from their usual social support in a time of crisis.[74]

In addition to the care provided to individual residents, the palliative care nurses and team supported the implementation of systemic approaches to support comfort and well-being in residents. The team brainstormed with staff to develop a tool to measure and track baseline function and promote activity and "new normal" activities of daily routine. Residents who qualified for a restorative plan of care were formally admitted to home care. Those who were at risk for deconditioning participated in exercises in their rooms; some followed exercise instruction via a closed-circuit television channel. The team worked with the facilities' dietary staff to provide fluids on each floor that could be offered between meals. Because residents missed the socialization and ambience of communal meals, staff members sat in the room with residents to socialize during meals and replated the meal from Styrofoam onto the resident's own dinnerware. Intake and output sheets were posted so that poor intake could be identified and addressed. Residents who were COVID-positive often deteriorated rapidly and were provided hospicelike care, including bereavement support to other residents, staff, and families.[74]

Even with the support of external services agencies and services, COVID-19 has presented ongoing challenges for assisted living to maintain resident quality of life. Notably, there have been more than 44,000 additional deaths due to dementia since February 1, 2020.[75] Experts opine that this statistic underscores a need for attention to resident health and quality of life and the integration of more, consistent psychosocial and medical care into ALs. This type of progress would need to be informed by research on different models of integrated, interdisciplinary health care that engage relevant stakeholders including residents, families, staff, administrators, and regulators in their development and evaluation.[76]

Adult Day Services

Adult day services provide a planned program offered in a group setting for older adults and persons with disabilities that offers social activities, meals, and health care monitoring. Services offered can vary; some provide case management, complex nursing care, rehabilitation, and caregiver training.[6] Adult day services also provide respite and relief to family caregivers so they can work or attend to other responsibilities and self-care needs. The programs are staffed by nurses, social workers, health aides, activity professionals, and other health professionals such as rehabilitation therapists. As of 2016, there were 4600 adult day programs serving approximately 286,300 older adults throughout the United States.[9] The predominant payer is Medicaid (66%).[77] The Veterans Administration is the second largest public source of reimbursement. Medicare does not pay for adult day services. Some participants pay out of pocket for care and even fewer use LTC insurance to pay for care.[78]

Participants in adult day services tend to have a high prevalence of chronic health conditions that have been associated with risk for severe illness from COVID-19 such as hypertension, diabetes, or dementia.[4,77] Because of their multiple comorbidities, many clients who attend adult day services would be eligible for nursing home level care, yet because of their preferences to age-in-place they remain in the community and use adult day services. The COVID-19 pandemic forced ADS to close and abruptly end in-person services to clients. Most of them were closed due to a state mandate.[79,80] In a national survey, sites continued to provide included telephone support (n = 22, 100%), delivery of food (n = 8, 36.4%), medical check-ins (n = 9, 40.1%), and activity via Zoom or YouTube (n = 14, 63.6%). Most of these services were provided without reimbursement. In these cases, nurses and other staff and administrators volunteered their time demonstrating extraordinary commitment to their clients. In some states, Medicaid waivers covered reimbursement for daily telephonic wellness check-ins, on-line social and activities, and care-coordination services.[81] An important lesson offered by the experience of adult day services is the valuable contribution of remote and flexible services offered during the pandemic. Future research is warranted that examines the clinical efficacy and cost-effectiveness of reimbursing these services.

SUMMARY

The needs of older adults admitted to LTC settings are increasingly complex. The COVID-19 pandemic has highlighted the need to not only prepare for crises but also respond with nurse-led care and services that are person-centered, family-engaged, and support interdisciplinary collaboration. Furthermore, models of care need to incorporate a comprehensive commitment to function and well-being—physical, social, and emotional—of older adults, their families, and staff.[82]

CLINICS CARE POINTS

- The infection preventionist (IP) nurse is an essential role to track cases of infection, educate staff, oversee testing, and monitor facility infection prevention and control practices.
- The unintended consequences of restricted visitation and isolation practices for residents include depression, anxiety, delirium, nutritional problems, symptoms of psychological distress, delirium, and functional decline.
  - Nursing interventions include encouraging regular family contact via telephone or video messages and recorded video messages from family/friends.
  - Structured, consistent rounding to provide cognitive stimulation and social interaction, snacks and fluids, and physical activity help prevent delirium and functional decline.
  - Sit-to-stand exercises, walking, and encouragement of self-care in hygiene and grooming can be incorporated into rounds and room visitations.
- Trauma-informed resident care includes knowing the person, looking for the reason behind behaviors, acting with empathy, engaging the person's social support, and providing choices.
- Strategies to support staff well-being include ensuring sufficient supply of equipment, consistent assignments, and clear, solid communication from supervisors, staff huddles that allow pause, acknowledging staff contributions, celebrating resident recoveries, and highlighting recognition from patients and families.

DISCLOSURE

The authors have nothing to disclose.

REFERENCES

1. National Center for Health Statistics. Provisional death counts for coronavirus disease. Washington, DC: National Center for Health Statistics; 2020. Available at: https://www.cdc.gov/nchs/nvss/vsrr/covid19/index.htm. Accessed June 24, 2022.

2. Belanger T. The coronavirus is killing too many nursing home residents. New York Times. Kaiser Family Foundation. State Health Facts: Total Number of Residents in Certified Nursing Facilities. 2020. Available at. https://www.kff.org/other/state-indicator/number-of-nursing-facility-residents/?. Accessed June 22, 2022.

3. Bakerjian D. Coronavirus disease 2019 (COVID-19) and safety of older adults. Agency for Healthcare Research and Quality Patient Safety Network. Available at. https://psnet.ahrq.gov/index.php/primer/coronavirus-disease-2019-covid-19-and-safety-older-adults#. Accessed June 27, 2022.

4. Centers for Disease Control and Prevention. Nursing Home Covid-19 Data Dashboard Nursing Homes Data Dashboard | NHSN | CDC. Available at: https://www.cdc.gov/nhsn/covid19/ltc-vaccination-dashboard.html. Accessed June 26, 2022.

5. Yi SH, See I, Kent AG, et al. Characterization of COVID-19 in Assisted Living Facilities - 39 States, October. MMWR Morbidity Mortality Weekly Report 2020; 69(46):1730–5.

6. Gaugler J, Marx JE, Dabelko-Schoeny H, et al. COVID-19 and the Need for Adult Day Services. J Am Med Dir Assoc 2021;22(7):1333–7. https://doi.org/10.1016/j.jamda.2021.04.025.

7. Kreitzer MJ. Voices of Nurses During the Covid-19 Pandemic: A Call to Action. Creat Nurs 2021;27(2):88–93. https://doi.org/10.1891/CRNR-D-21-00005.

8. US Government Accountability Office COVID-19 in Nursing Homes: Most Homes Had Multiple Outbreaks and Weeks of Sustained Transmission from May 2020 through January 2021 | U.S. GAO. 2021. Available at: https://www.gao.gov/products/gao-21-367. Accessed June 26, 2022.

9. Harris-Kojetin L, Sengupta M, Lendon JP, et al. Long-term care providers and services users in the United States, 2015–2016. Natl Cent Health Stat Vital Health Stat 3(43) 2019.

10. Vincent Mor V, Angelelli J, Teno JM, et al. Driven to Tiers: Socioeconomic and Racial Disparities in the Quality of Nursing Home Care. Milbank Q 2004;82(2): 227–56.

11. Harrington C, Ross L, Chapman S, et al. Nursing staffing and coronavirus infections in California NHs. Pol Polit Nurs Pract 2020;21(2):174–86.

12. Li Y, Temkin-Greener H, Shan G, et al. COVID- 19 infections and deaths among Connecticut nursing home residents: facility correlates. J Am Geriatr Soc 2020; 68(9):1899–906. https://doi.org/10.1111/jgs.16689.

13. Wiliams CS, Qing Z, White AJ, et al. The association of nursing home quality ratings and spread of COVID-19. J Am Geriatr Soc 2021;69(8):2070–8. https://doi.org/10.1111/jgs.17309.

14. Bui DP, Isaac See I, Hesse EM, et al. Association Between CMS Quality Ratings and COVID-19 Outbreaks in Nursing Homes - West Virginia. MMWR Morb Mortal Wkly Rep 2020;69(37):1300–4.

15. Abrams HR, Loomer L, Gandhi A, et al. Characteristics of U.S. Nursing Homes with COVID-19 Cases. J Am Geriatr Soc 2020;68(8):1653–6.

16. Mendoza A. Facility Location Determines COVID Outbreaks, Researchers Say. Provider 5/12/2020.

17. Bagchi S, Mak J, Li Qunna. Rates of COVID-19 Among Residents and Staff Members in Nursing Homes — United States, May 25–November 22, 2020 | MMWR (cdc.gov).

18. Panagiotou OA, Cyrus M, Kosar CM, et al. Risk Factors Associated With All-Cause 30-Day Mortality in Nursing Home Residents With COVID-19. JAMA Intern Med 2021;181(4):439–48. https://doi.org/10.1001/jamainternmed.2020.7968.

19. Testimony of R. Tamara Konetzka. Available at: www.SCA_Konetzka_05_21_20.pdf (senate.gov). Accessed: June 22, 2022.

20. Dosa D, Jump RLP, LaPlante K, et al. Long-term care facilities and the coronavirus epidemic: practical guidelines for a population at highest risk. J Am Med Dir Assoc 2020. https://doi.org/10.1016/j.jamda.2020.03.004.

21. Giri S, Lee MC, Romero-Ortuno R. Nursing homes during the COVID-19 pandemic: a scoping review of challenges and responses. Eur Geriatr Med 2021;12:1127–36.

22. Bakerjian D, Boltz M, Bowers B, et al. Expert nurse response to workforce recommendations made by The Coronavirus Commission For Safety And Quality In Nursing Homes. Nurs Outlook 2021;69(5):735–43. https://doi.org/10.1016/j.outlook.2021.03.017.

23. Kolanowski A, Cortes TA, Mueller C, et al. A call to the CMS: Mandate adequate professional nurse staffing in nursing homes. Am J Nurs 2021;121:24–7.

24. Center for Medicare and Medicaid Services. Final Rule-81 FR 68688. Available at: https://www.federalregister.gov/documents/2016/10/04/2016-23503/medicare-and-medicaid-programs-reform-of-requirements-for-long-term-care-facilities. Accessed June 26, 2022.

25. Rubano MD, Kieffer EF, Larson EL. Infection prevention and control in nursing homes during COVID-19: An environmental scan. Geriatr Nurs 2022;43:51–7.

26. Agarwal M, Dick A, Sorbero M, et al. Changes in US nursing home infection prevention and control programs from 2014 to 2018. J Am Med Dir Assoc 2020; 21(1). https://doi.org/10.1016/j.jamda.2019.10.020.

27. Stone P, Agarwal M, Pogorzelska-Maziarz M. Infection preventionist staffing in nursing homes. Am J Infect Control 2020;48(3). https://doi.org/10.1016/j.ajic.2019.12.010.

28. Chan GK, Waxman KT, Baggett M, et al. The Importance and Impact of Nurse Leader Engagement With State Nursing Workforce Centers: Lessons From the COVID-19 Pandemic. Nurse Leader 2021;19(6):576–80.

29. Commission for Safety and Quality in Nursing Homes. Available at: https://sites.mitre.org/nhcovidcomm/. Accessed: June 28, 2002.

30. Silverstein W, Kowalski M. Adapting a professional practice model. Am Nurse Today 2017;12(9):78–83.

31. Abbasi J. Social isolation—the other COVID-19 threat in nursing homes. JAMA 2020;324(7):619–20.

32. Hwang T-J, Rabheru K, Peisah C, et al. Loneliness and social isolation during the COVID-19 pandemic. Int Psychogeriatrics 2020;32:1217–20.

33. Chu CH, Donato-Woodger S, Dainton CJ. Competing crises: COVID-19 countermeasures and social isolation among older adults in long-term care. J Adv Nurs 2020;76(10):2456–9.

34. Chu CH, Wang J, Fukui C, et al. The Impact of COVID-19 on Social isolation in long-term care homes: Perspectives of policies and strategies from six countries. J Aging Social Policy 2021;33(4–5):459–73.

35. El Haj M, Altintas E, Chapelet G, et al. High depression and anxiety in people with Alzheimer's disease living in retirement homes during the -19 crisis. Psychiatry Res 2020. 291, Article 113294.

36. O' Caoimh R, O'Donovan MR, Monahan MP,O'Connor CD, et al. Psychosocial Impact of COVID-19 nursing home restrictions on visitors of residents with cognitive impairment: A cross-sectional study as part of the Engaging Remotely in Care (ERiC) project. Front Psychiatry 2020;2020(11):585373.

37. Simard J, Volicer L. Loneliness and isolation in long-term care and the COVID-19 pandemic. J Am Med Dir Assoc 2020;21(7):966–7.

38. Martinchek M, Beiting JK, Walker J, et al. Weight Loss in COVID-19- Positive Nursing Home Residents. Research Letters. J Am Med Dir Assoc 2021;22: 256e262.

39. Danilovich MK, Norrick CR, Hill KC, et al. Nursing home resident weight loss during coronavirus disease 2019 restrictions. J Am Med Dir Assoc 2020;21(11): 1568–9.

40. Sweeney MR, Boilson A, White S, et al. Experiences of residents, family members and staff in residential care settings for older people during COVID-19: A mixed methods study. J Nurs Manag 2022;30(4):872–82.

41. Bethell J, Aelick K, Babineau J, et al. Social connection in long- term care homes: A scoping review of published research on the mental health impacts and potential strategies during COVID-19. J Am Med Dir Assoc 2021;22:228–37.

42. Bolt SR, van der Steen JT, Mujezinovoc I, et al. Practical nursing recommendations for palliative care for people with dementia living in long-term care facilities during the COVID-19 pandemic: A rapid scoping review. Int J Nurs Stud 2021; 113:103781.

43. Tsai HH, Tsai YF, Wang HH, et al. Videoconference program enhances social support, loneliness, and depressive status of elderly nursing home residents. Aging Ment Health 2010;14:947e954.

44. Gorenko JA, Moran C, Flynn M, et al. Social isolation and psychological distress among older adults related to COVID-19: a narrative review of remotely-delivered interventions and recommendations. J Appl Gerontol 2021;40(1):3–13.

45. Noone C, McSharry J, Smalle M, et al. Video calls for reducing social isolation and loneliness in older people: a rapid review. Cochrane Database 2020.

46. Jacobs M, Ellis C. Telemedicine disparities during COVID-19: provider offering and individual technology availability. J Am Geriatr Soc 2021;69:2432e2434.

47. Savage R, Rochon P, Na Y, et al. Excess mortality in long-term care residents with and without personal contact with family or friends during the COVID-19 pandemic. J Am Med Dir Assoc 2022;23:441e443.e1.

48. Seifert A, Batsis JA, Smith AC. Telemedicine in long-term care facilities during and beyond COVID-19: challenges caused by the digital divide. Front Public Health 2020;8:601595.

49. Vu T, Frye N, Valeika S, et al. Communication Technology Improved Staff, Resident, and Family Interactions in a Skilled Nursing Home During COVID-19. JAMDA 23 2022;947e953.

50. Havaei F, Macphee M, Keselman D, et al. Leading a long-term care facility through the COVID-19 crisis: successes, barriers and lessons learned. Health Q 2021;23(4):28–34.

51. Chow L. Care homes and COVID-19 in Hong Kong: how the lessons from SARS were used to good effect. Age Ageing 2021;50(1):21–4.

52. Chu CH, Quan A, Gandhi F, et al. Person-centered physical activity for nursing home residents with dementia: The perspectives of family members and care staff. Health Expect 2021. https://doi.org/10.1111/hex.13381.

53. Aubertin-Leheudre M, Rolland Y. The importance of physical activity to care for frail older adults during the COVID-19 pandemic. J Am Med Dir Assoc 2020; 21(7):973–6. https://doi.org/10.1016/j.jamda.2020.04.022.

54. Canevelli M, Bruno G, Cesari M. Providing simultaneous COVID-19-sensitive and dementia-sensitive care as we transition from crisis care to ongoing care. J Am Med Dir Assoc 2020;21(7):968–9. https://doi.org/10.1016/j.jamda.2020.05.025.

55. Levenson S. Trauma-Informed Care and Regulatory Expectations. Caring for the Ages 2022;23(2):8–9.

56. SAMHSA's Trauma and Justice Strategic Initiative, Concept of Trauma and Guidance for Trauma Informed Care Approach, HHS Publication No. (SMA) 14-4884, July 2014. Available at: https://bit.ly/3AqbMKY. Accessed: June 36, 2022.

57. Desai A, Grossberg G. Psychiatric consultation in long-term care. 2nd edition. Cambridge University Press; 2017.

58. Beausoleil F. Best Practices for Increasing Compassion Resiliency and Moral Wellness in Post-Acute and Long-Term Care Settings. Caring for the Ages 2022;23(2):12–3.

59. Chan D, Livingston G, Jones L, et al. Grief reactions in dementia carers: a systematic review. Int J Geriatr Psychiatry 2013;28(1):1–17.

60. Sjostrom S. Turning the Lens of Trauma-Informed Care Toward Staff with Stress First Aid. Sjostrom Caring for the Ages 2022;23(2):12–3.

61. Lateef FJ. Face to Face with Coronavirus Disease 19: Maintaining Motivation, Psychological Safety, and Wellness. Emerg Trauma Shock 2020;13(2):116–23.

62. Kilpatrick K, Tchouaket É, Jabbour M, et al. A mixed methods quality improvement study to implement nurse practitioner roles and improve care for residents in long-term care facilities. BMC Nurs 2020;19:6. https://doi.org/10.1186/s12912-019-0395-2.

63. Popejoy L, Vogelsmeier A, Galambos C, et al. The APRN role in changing nursing home quality: the Missouri quality improvement initiative. J Nurs Care Qual 2017; 32(3):196–201.

64. Vogelsmeier A, Popejoy L, Galambos C, et al. Results of the Missouri quality initiative in sustaining changes in nursing home care: six-year trends of reducing hospitalizations of nursing home residents. J Nutr Health Aging 2021;25(1):5–12.

65. Kane RL, Keckhafer G, Flood S, et al. The effect of Evercare on hospital use. J Am Geriatr Soc 2003;51(10):1427–34.

66. McGilton KS, Krassikova A, Boscart V, et al. Nurse Practitioners Rising to the Challenge During the Coronavirus Disease 2019 Pandemic in Long-Term Care Homes. Gerontologist 2021;61(4):615–23.

67. Vellani S, Boscart V, Escrig-Pinol A, et al. Complexity of Nurse Practitioners' Role in Facilitating a Dignified Death for Long-Term Care Home Residents during the COVID-19 Pandemic. J Pers Med 2021;433:11.

68. Kleinpell R, Myers CR, Schorn MN, et al. Impact of COVID-19 pandemic on APRN practice: Results from a national survey. Nurs Outlook 2021;69(5):783–92.

69. Bakerjian D. The Advanced Practice Registered Nurse Leadership Role in Nursing Homes Leading Efforts Toward High Quality and Safe Care. Nurs Clin N Am 2022;57:245–58.

70. Yee-Melichar D, Flores C, Boyle AR. Assisted living administration and management. New York: Springer; 2021.

71. American Geriatrics Society. American Geriatrics Society (AGS) Policy Brief: COVID-19 and Assisted Living Facilities. J Am Geriatr Soc 2020;68(6):1131–5.
72. Terebuh PD, Egwiekhor AJ, Gullett HL, et al. Characterization of community-wide transmission of SARS-CoV-2 in congregate living settings and local public health-coordinated response during the initial phase of the COVID-19 pandemic. Influenza other Respir viruses 2021;15(4):439–45.
73. Dobbs D, Peterson L, Hyer K. The Unique Challenges Faced by Assisted Living Communities to Meet Federal Guidelines for COVID-19. J Aging Social Policy 2020;32(4–5):334–42.
74. de Campos AP, Daniels S. Ethical implications of COVID-19: Palliative care, public health, and long-term care facilities. J Hosp Palliat Nurs 2021;23:120–7.
75. Centers for Disease Control and Prevention. Excess deaths associated with COVID-19. Available at: https://www.cdc.gov/nchs/nvss/vsrr/covid19/excess_.deaths.htm. Accessed June 26, 2022.
76. Vipperman A, Zimmerman S, Sloane PD. COVID-19 Recommendations for Assisted Living: Implications for the Future. J Am Med Dir Assoc 2021;22(5):933–8.e5.
77. Parker LJ, Marx K, Gaugler JE, et al. Implications of the COVID-19 Pandemic on Adult Day Services and the Families They Serve. Am J Alzheimers Dis Other Demen 2021;36. 15333175211050152.
78. Harris-Kojetin L, Sengupta M, Lendon JP. Long-term care providers and services users in the United States, 2015–2016. National Center for Health Statistics. Vital Health Stat. 2019;3.
79. Anderson KA, Dabelko-Schoeny H, Fields NL, editors. Home and community-based Services for older adults: Aging in Context. New York, NY: Columbia University Press; 2018.
80. Sands LP, Albert SM, Suitor JJ. Understanding and addressing older adults' needs during COVID-19. Innov Aging 2020;4(3). igaa019.
81. Caffrey C, Lendon JP. Service provision, hospitalizations, and chronic conditions in adult day services centers: Findings from the 2016 national study of long-term care providers. Natl Health Stat Rep 2019;124(124):1–9.
82. National Academy of Medicine. Strategies to Support the Health and Well-Being of Clinicians During COVID-19-National Academy of Medicine (nam.edu). Available at: Strategies to Support the Health and Well-Being of Clinicians During COVID-19-National Academy of Medicine (nam.edu) Accessed: June 27, 2022.

Preparing New Nurses During a Pandemic

Michael M. Evans, PhD, MSEd, RN, ACNS, CMSRN, CNE[a,*],
Kimberly Streiff, DEd, MSN, CCRN, CRNP, FNP-C[b], Catherine Stiller, PhD, RN, CNE[c],
Jennifer Barton, DNP, RN, CNE, WHNP-BC[d], Kiernan Riley, PhD, RN[e],
Kalei Kowalchik, BSN, RN[f]

KEYWORDS

- COVID-19 • Virtual learning • Innovation • Nursing • Nursing students
- Undergraduate nursing programs • Clinical

KEY POINTS

- When coordinating undergraduate nursing students' educational needs during times of emergency, administrators and nursing educators must address students' mental health and well-being.
- Throughout the COVID-19 pandemic, nursing educators and administrators across the world have had to integrate innovative learning resources to help meet the educational and learning needs of undergraduate nursing students.
- When given the opportunity to select in-person or virtual clinical opportunities during COVID-19 pandemic, undergraduate nursing students thought they made the best decision for them based on their physical or psychosocial needs.
- During the COVID-19 pandemic, student engagement with faculty and peers through zoom can foster classroom intimacy, socialization, and support, as well as develop thought-provoking discussions and clinical reasoning.

The authors have no financial or commercial conflicts of interest to disclose.
[a] The Pennsylvania State University, Ross and Carol Nese College of Nursing, Scranton Campus, 120 Ridge View Drive, Dunmore, PA 18512, USA; [b] The Pennsylvania State University, Ross and Carol Nese College of Nursing, Erie, The Behrend College, 11630 Lay Road, Edinboro, PA 16412, USA; [c] The Pennsylvania State University, Ross and Carol Nese College of Nursing, Erie, The Behrend College, 1704 Charles Street, Erie, PA 16509, USA; [d] The Pennsylvania State University, Ross and Carol Nese College of Nursing, Hershey Campus, 1300 ASB / A110, 90 Hope Drive, Hershey, PA 17033, USA; [e] Fitchburg State University, 412 Grafton Street, Worcester, MA 01604, USA; [f] The Pennsylvania State University, Ross and Carol Nese College of Nursing, University Park Campus, Nursing Sciences Building, University Park, PA 16802
* Corresponding author.
E-mail address: mme124@psu.edu

0029-6465/23/© 2022 Elsevier Inc. All rights reserved.

PREPARING NEW NURSES DURING A PANDEMIC

The coronavirus pandemic was declared by the World Health Organization on March 11, 2020. By April of 2020, most states reported widespread cases of COVID-19.[1] During the COVID-19 pandemic, most public spaces including university's in-person spaces were closed across the United States and worldwide to prevent the further spread of disease.[2] Nurse educators had to pivot immediately to provide didactic and clinical education in an online format to meet state and federal requirements to limit person-to-person contact.[3] Several strategies were developed to foster student engagement and to provide high-quality, educational experiences at multiple sites at a large research university in the form of emergency, remote in-person education using digital platforms such as Zoom and previous tools developed through Assessment Technologies Incorporated (ATI). The purpose of this article is to explore 2 exemplars of how educators transformed the undergraduate nursing educational experience to provide quality learning experiences to undergraduate prelicensure students in the remote environment.

BACKGROUND

Traditional prelicensure, nursing curricula heavily rely on in-person class and clinical activities; however, many programs were forced to switch to emergency, remote teaching due to the pandemic, a modality first described by Hodges and colleagues (2020).[4] Emergency, remote teaching is described as the temporary use of remote teaching strategies for a course that was intended to have an in-person component, either a blended course or fully in-person course. The key differences between emergency remote teaching and online teaching are the rationale for the delivery method—crisis or intentional design and future plans for the course—*will it return to face-to-face instruction once the crisis is over or will it remain an online course?*[4]

Johnson (2019) discusses that while temporary disruptions in educational delivery methods are not new, such disruptions have historically been limited to small regional areas for reasons such as political unrest or natural disasters.[5] Before COVID-19 disruptions in March 2020, few publications addressed the potential effect of a global pandemic on higher education. In the span of 2 months, March 2020 to May 2020, publications began appearing in the gray literature discussing many different aspects of emergency remote teaching in nursing education.[6,7] However, the speed with which the crisis unfolded meant there were no formal studies of emergency remote teaching for faculty to reference and implement into their nursing programs. Thus, nursing leadership had to make decisions based on current science to ensure the safety of their students while also allowing opportunities for students to meet course and clinical objectives and progress in the program. The following exemplars will describe 2 different initiatives used at this University: one involving the decisions that students made to continue their education in an in-person format or an all-virtual format during the COVID-19 pandemic and the other involving the transition of a course with a laboratory/clinical component to an all-online environment.

EXEMPLAR #1

In response to public health recommendations to help curb the spread of the emerging COVID-19 pandemic, a large research university in the mid-Atlantic part of the country transitioned to full-remote learning in March of 2020. By August of 2020, nursing students had mostly returned to in-person learning for both didactic and clinical courses. Shortly after returning, local campus factors, including an increase in students contracting or being exposed to COVID-19 at 1 of our 11 campuses, necessitated the implementation of transmission mitigation efforts that were more restrictive than other campuses within our system. These transmission mitigation efforts included:

- No overnight travel for students
- No travel beyond a 30-mile radius of campus
- No visitors in the students' homes
- No patronizing indoor bars or restaurants
- No attendance at any event/venue/business that was indoors
- Strict masking whenever the student left their homes

Students were, therefore, given a choice of remaining in person and adhering to the new mitigation requirements or going fully remote for class and clinical activities. Because a sizeable percentage, 38% in fall semester and 22% in the spring semester, opted to switch to virtual learning, this descriptive qualitative study was developed to gain a better understanding of the factors that influenced student decision-making.

METHODS

A qualitative survey design was utilized to explore student decision-making processes and experiences. The survey, developed by 4 of the researchers of this article, consisted of 5 (out of a possible 8) open-ended questions. Questions were logically provided to students based on their clinical choice: in-person or online. The survey questions with logic are shown in **Fig. 1**.

Following institutional review board approval, students who were third and fourth year standing at the campus were purposively sampled via email. The survey was entered into Qualtrics online software, and the link was distributed via email to eligible students by a person not related to the research so students would not feel coerced to complete the survey. Students had approximately 1-month to complete the online survey. The choice to fill out the online survey implied consent.

Following data collection, data analysis of the transcript occurred. Thematic analysis techniques and descriptive analysis techniques were applied by 2 researchers and verified with the research team.

RESULTS

Of the 150 potential student participants, 26 students answered the anonymous survey for a return rate of approximately 17%. The sample included 26 third-year and fourth-year undergraduate student participants from the host university. Several of the participants (n = 17) chose to engage in an in-person clinical format during the Spring 2021 semester, whereas other participants (n = 9) chose virtual clinical format.

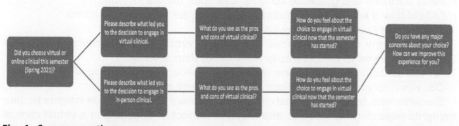

Fig. 1. Survey questions.

Research questions 1 and 2 were evaluated using a thematic analysis, where responses were reviewed by multiple authors for patterns throughout the data. Research questions 3 through 8 were reviewed using a descriptive analysis based on the format of the questions.

Results by Research Question

Q1: *Please describe what led you to decision to engage in virtual clinical.*

Participant's answers varied in response and included themes such as fear of social isolation, and the impact of nonacademic commitments.

Exemplar quotes used to support student's expression of fear of isolation include: "*…campus wasn't allowed to go places (social outings), it wasn't a good option for me mentally.*"

Another participant stated.

"*…I had to decide if I wanted my mental health to decline from social isolation and not be able to work or attend in-person clinicals and not have the option to leave for work.*"

Some students described the importance of having virtual clinical experiences during their final semester of their undergraduate education.

"*Although it wasn't hands on clinical, I still learned critical thinking skills and was able to enjoy what was left of my senior year rather than being upset and depressed like I was in the fall semester.*"

Some students describe the nonacademic commitments they were able to pursue because they selected to engage in virtual clinical:

"*Enabling access and participation in commitments and relationships out of …[the host university].*"

"*I didn't think it would impact my career long-term.*"

Q2: *Please describe what led you to the choice to engage in an in-person clinical.*

Many participants rationalized their choice to selecting an in-person clinical experience. Themes emerged regarding having trust in the traditional learning experience as well as many feared that the virtual environment would not be substantial to meet their learning and professional needs.

Some students described that they were comfortable with the traditional, in-person clinical experiences provided to them and thought that being in-person was the only way to adequately obtain those skills. Participants stated:

"*I did not want to miss out on hands on experiences.*"

"*Online clinical could never replace the experience felt by in-person clinical.*"

"*I felt that in-person clinical was an invaluable experience. Being in-person has helped me learn skills such as confidence, flexibility, communication skills, etc. that cannot be learned virtually.*"

Additionally, students thought that participating in in-person clinical settings would be the best opportunity to develop their nursing skills because they began applying for nursing positions and graduate schools. Exemplar quotes included:

"*Afraid how it would look on future job or graduate school applications.*"

"*I knew that I needed it for my future.*"

"*Based on my own experiences of personal, virtual clinical experience from Fall 2020; there seems to be more busy work rather than learning.*"

"*Virtual simulations do not allow me to feel confident in my nursing skills.*"

Q3: *What do you see as the Pros and Cons of virtual clinical?*

Students who selected a virtual clinical format were able to provide insights to their thoughts regarding the positive and negative aspect of engaging in a virtual clinical experience. Although there were some negative aspects highlighted, a majority of comments surrounded positive takeaways students perceived through participating in virtual clinical as showcased in **Table 1**.

Q4: *What do you see as the Pros and Cons of in-person clinical?*

Students who selected to participate in an in-person clinical format were able to describe their thoughts about the pros and cons of selecting to be in-person for their clinical experiences. Although participants enjoyed the ability to develop their nursing skills and engage with faculty and peers, some students thought that social isolation and the risks of being in-person were drawbacks to their clinical experiences as described in **Table 2**.

Q5: *How do you feel about the decision to engage in virtual clinical now that the semester has started?*

Several participants described their thoughts surrounding their decision to partake in a virtual clinical format while they were participating in their clinical experiences. Students provided a variety of personalized responses, with most of them providing positive responses about their decision, including:

- *"It was the right decision for me."*
- *"I don't regret it."*
- *"Virtual clinical allowed me to improve my critical thinking."*
- *"Virtual clinical has enabled me to understand how diseases work and why certain treatments are beneficial. I can always re-learn or practice skills."*

Q6: *How do you feel about the decision to engage in an in-person clinical now that the semester has started?*

Many students detailed their decision of selecting an in-person clinical experience. Participants provided multiple mixed responses regarding their decision to participate in an in-person clinical experience, such as follows:

- *"I feel like I made the right decision."*
- *"I am glad I did it for the hands-on learning, but I would probably be at a better place mentally if I chose virtual."*
- *"I have had valuable in person clinical experiences, so I am happy with my decision."*

Q7: *Do you have any major concerns about your choice? How can we improve this experience for you?*

All participants had the opportunity to discuss any concerns regarding their decision to select an in-person or virtual clinical experience. Participants described concerns such as marketability, social experiences, development of nursing skills, and the impact their clinical choice has on mental health and wellness. Exemplar quotes include

- *"Biggest concern is that when applying for jobs people won't perceive virtual clinical as well as in-person clinical."*
- *"My major concern is that I am missing out time with my friends."*
- *"I am concerned if I am still on track with my peers."*
- *"By staying remote I have missed out on skills I should have learned."*
- *"Severe COVID-19 restrictions have made my experience undesirable."*
- *"This has substantially and negatively impacted my mental health (in person)."*
- *"There needs to be more open communication with students from administration and not just them telling us what we are and aren't going to do."*
- *"I feel it was a good choice for me and I was given adequate resources to succeed virtually."*

Table 1	
Pros and cons of virtual clinical	
The Pros of Virtual Clinical	**The Cons of Virtual Clinical**
Allows time to be home with family Less stress Provides time to apply for graduate nurse positions	Poor opportunities for hands-on experiences
Offers time for students to focus on their personal health and wellness Creates more time allotted for critical thinking	Unable to participate in therapeutic communication at the bedside
Provides students access to use case studies and understand deeper learning of nursing practice	Lack of live patient interactions

- *"I just wished students were able to care for COVID-19 positive patients—we will have to in a few months in the real world."*

CONCLUSION AND IMPLICATIONS

Shortly after returning to full in-person learning, campus administrators were faced with an outbreak of COVID-19 among a relatively close population of students. In working with the health department, epidemiologists, and infectious disease experts, the decision was made to implement notably restrictive mitigation efforts. Throughout the discussions and decision-making process, administrators had one main goal—prevent further transmission of COVID-19 to the wider campus community while minimizing the educational impact to the affected students, which was achieved because this University's NCLEX-RN scores remained above 92%. The results of this study show that students had another main goal that was not considered by administrators as much as it maybe—minimizing the effect of the resultant social isolation that would influence students' mental health and well-being.

The effects of social isolation and loneliness are documented as having significant effects among students, and nursing students are no exception. Labrague, De los Santos, and Falguera (2020) found high levels of loneliness among a sample of Philippine nursing students who were affected by mandatory lockdown orders; students who were younger and identified as women were more likely to experience loneliness

Table 2	
Pros and cons of in-person clinical	
The Pros of In-Person Clinical	**The Cons of In-Person Clinical**
Can participate in hands-on care	Risk of potential COVID-19 exposure
Ability to participate in in-person classrooms with faculty and peers	Limited specialty, clinical experiences available (eg, lack of neonatal intensive care unit [NICIU] opportunities)
Provides an opportunity to develop therapeutic communication skills	Sacrificing ability to see family due to restrictions placed by host university (eg, unable to travel home weekly)
Offers time to develop self-confidence Can help to sustain a "normal-college" life/experience	Experiencing feelings of social isolation

because of the lockdown orders as opposed to those who were older and identified as men.[8] Factors that had a positive influence on loneliness were personal resilience, coping skills, and social support.[8]

These findings indicate how imperative it is for administrators and educators who are faced with implementing restrictive public health measures within their campus community to approach the problem with a holistic, student-centered mindset. Providing students with physical and educational safety during a public health crisis is not enough; steps must also be taken to help foster students' psychological safety as well such as providing them with national and campus-based psychosocial resources.

EXEMPLAR #2

The COVID-19 pandemic and the sequela of changes it has caused in higher education forced nurse educators to change their teaching styles in new and innovative ways.[6] Nursing faculty at a large research university in the mid-Atlantic region responded to the mitigation challenges of COVID-19 by transitioning a health assessment course to an all-virtual format. Therefore, the purpose of this study was to determine the efficacy of transitioning an undergraduate health assessment course for prelicensure baccalaureate nursing students from an in-person format to an all-virtual format.

METHODS

The faculty recognized the importance and value of maintaining high levels of engagement and delivering real-time feedback to the students while they practiced hands-on assessment skills. The structural integrity of the course was maintained as closely as possible, while transitioning from in-person instruction to an all-virtual format.

The assessment course had both a class and clinical component and with 58 second-year sophomore nursing students. Traditional pieces of the course that remained intact included the use of the course management system, CANVAS, the course content, and small laboratory sections of 6 to 8 students for skills practice with instructor feedback. The class continued to meet weekly in a virtual classroom for lecture content, which was delivered synchronously via Zoom. The clinical laboratory sections met at the regularly scheduled times where their laboratory instructor demonstrated physical assessment skills. This was augmented by video presentations, using Kaltura, and ATI learning modules including HealthAssess, Skills Modules 2.0, and Nurses Touch. Questions and interaction were encouraged in these sessions. Zoom technology allowed for pairing off of students or arranging students in small groups for learning content such as completing the general survey, or in practicing interviewing skills. Each week students were required to complete a system assessment demonstration on a peer, or family member using a feature of Canvas called Kaltura, which allowed videotaping of the presentation. The presentations were viewed by instructors weekly and feedback was posted.

RESULTS

Midsemester surveys were used to gather student feedback on the course and the transition of the course to a virtual format. Midsemester evaluations revealed student satisfaction. Some comments included:

- *"I actually like learning online. I am a visual learner, so what helps me most is videos that show what to do with assessments, and written directions, as well as PowerPoints explaining key concepts."*
- *"I like having the sample documentations and videos to help me get an idea of what things are supposed to look like because having a Zoom and no in-person lab can make things confusing at times."*
- *"I find that I learn best in this course from the engagement of polls on Zoom-it allows me to stay focused. I also find that I learn best from making the Kaltura videos and getting feedback on them."*

Ultimately, 96% of students passed the course, and 98% passed the clinical component.

LIMITATIONS

There were inherent limitations to this learning experience. Students were not exposed to variation in assessments because their assessment partners were limited to those who lived with them and they did not have expert hands on feedback as they would in a normal laboratory. To overcome these limitations, a boot camp was offered at the start of the Fall 2022 semester, which consisted of several days of focus sessions to help students feel more comfortable with their assessments. This proved beneficial because the majority of students were then able to transition back to in-person learning and were successful in their third-year class and clinical courses.

CONCLUSION AND IMPLICATIONS

The purpose of this study was to determine the efficacy of transitioning an undergraduate health assessment course for prelicensure baccalaureate nursing students from an in-person format to an all-virtual format. This study has shown that the use of technology to learn and practice assessment skills can be utilized effectively to meet course and clinical objectives. Additionally, the use of technology can standardize messages and clearly define expectations of the assessment skills to be demonstrated for student learning. Use of zoom technology afforded faculty the ability to witness firsthand skill acquisition and gave them the opportunity to provide real-time feedback to their students.

In times of social isolation, student engagement with faculty and with each other in the zoom classroom provides the intimacy that lends itself to a milieu of ongoing interaction and support. The use of virtual laboratories seems to lend itself to more thought-provoking discussion, which may enhance clinical reasoning for undergraduate prelicensure baccalaureate nursing students.

OVERALL CONCLUSIONS

Nursing faculty, similar to bedside nurses, proved to be innovative and resilient during the COVID-19 pandemic and continued to provide the best educational experiences possible for students. In addition, faculty learned new teaching/learning strategies that will continue to push nursing education forward and higher education in general. By continuing to provide high-quality nursing education, this university was able to graduate competent, novice nurses who were able to immediately provide care at the bedside during one of the nation's biggest crises. Moving forward, faculty and administrators must remain aware of the influence of COVID-19 on our students' mental health and ensure that resources are available to them.

CLINICS CARE POINTS

- Virtual learning in prelicensure nursing education has benefits including more time for students to understand concepts and engage in clinical reasoning skills; however, faculty and administrators must be cognizant of students' mental health and well-being.

- Various nursing education vendors provide resources to enhance online learning experiences and should be considered when developing teaching strategies for courses; however, hands on practice still needs to be implemented.

- Nurse educators and administrators should consider the benefits of hybrid learning opportunities moving forward to provide students with both virtual and in-person learning experiences.

REFERENCES

1. CDC Museum Covid-19 Timeline. Centers for Disease Control and Prevention. 2022. Available at: https://www.cdc.gov/museum/timeline/covid19.html. Accessed June 26, 2022.
2. Yu HJ, Hu YF, Liu XX, et al. Household infection: The predominant risk factor for close contacts of patients with COVID-19. Travel Med Infect Dis 2020;36:101809.
3. Rafael RMR, Correia LM, Mello AS, et al. Psychological distress in the COVID-19 pandemic: prevalence and associated factors at a nursing college. Rev Bras Enferm 2021;74. https://doi.org/10.1590/0034-7167-2021-0023.
4. Hodges C, Moore S, Trust T, et al. The difference between emergency remote teaching and online learning. 2020. Available at: https://er.educause.edu/articles/2020/3/the-difference-between-emergency-remote-teaching-and-online-learning. Accessed June 26, 2022.
5. Johnson E. As fires rage, more campuses close. 2019. Available at: https://www.insidehighered.com/news/2019/10/29/california-fires-and-power-outages-close-campuses; https://www.insidehighered.com/news/2019/10/29/california-fires-and-power-outages-close-campuses. Accessed June 26, 2020.
6. Dewart G, Corcoran L, Thirsk L, et al. Nursing education in a pandemic: Academic challenges in response to COVID-19. Nurse Educ Today 2020;92:104471.
7. Morin K. Nursing education after COVID-19: Same or different. J Clin Nurs 2020; 29(17–18):17–9.
8. Labrague LJ, De Los Santos JAA, Falguera CC. Social and emotional loneliness among college students during the COVID-19 pandemic: The predictive role of coping behaviors, social support, and personal resilience. Perspect Psychiatr Care 2021;57(4):1578–84.

Diversity Impacts of Coronavirus Disease 2019

Sarah Hexem Hubbard, JD[a],*, Jennifer Gimbel, MBA[b], Zaharaa Davood, MPH[b], Monica Harmon, MSN, MPH, RN[c]

KEYWORDS

- Diversity • Cultural competence • Belonging • COVID-19 • Mentorship • Podcast
- Nursing • Workforce

KEY POINTS

- The COVID-19 pandemic highlighted the impact of systemic oppression on communities of color concurrent with and inextricable from the national reckoning with racism in 2020.
- The *Future of Nursing* reports and their implementation through the activities of the *Campaign for Action* and state Action Coalitions exemplify strategies to connect macro-level concepts and research with targeted activities.
- Mentorship is a key component of efforts to bolster a diverse nursing workforce.
- Coalition work leverages the strength of diversity, including across sectors, disciplines, professions, and backgrounds.
- Podcasting is an emerging modality for disseminating information that continues to gain popularity.

 Video content accompanies this article at http://www.nursing.theclinics.com.

Three of the podcast episodes listed in this article were funded in part by a cooperative agreement with the Centers for Disease Control and Prevention (grant number NU50CK000580). The Centers for Disease Control and Prevention is an agency within the Department of Health and Human Services (HHS). The contents of this resource center do not necessarily represent the policy of CDC or HHS, and should not be considered an endorsement by the Federal Government.
[a] National Nurse-Led Care Consortium, 4601 Market Street, 2nd Floor, Philadelphia, PA 19139, USA; [b] National Nurse-Led Care Consortium - Pennsylvania Action Coalition, 4601 Market Street, 2nd Floor, Philadelphia, PA 19139, USA; [c] Drexel University, College of Nursing and Health Professions Community Wellness HUB, Pennsylvania Action Coalition, Nurse Diversity Council, Dornsife Center for Neighborhood Partnerships, Carriage House - Second Floor, 3509 Spring Garden Street, Philadelphia, PA 19104, USA
* Corresponding author.
E-mail address: shexem@phmc.org
Twitter: @sahexem (S.H.H.); @jenniferhorngim (J.G.); @MonicaJH21451 (M.H.)

Nurs Clin N Am 58 (2023) 59–75
https://doi.org/10.1016/j.cnur.2022.10.003
0029-6465/23/© 2022 Elsevier Inc. All rights reserved.

INTRODUCTION

The coronavirus disease 2019 (COVID-19) pandemic continues to underscore the need for a nursing workforce that reflects the diversity of the communities it serves and that is prepared to promote social justice. Although the COVID-19 virus was novel, its disparate impacts were not. The need for diversity and to better prepare nurses to meet the needs of diverse communities did not result from COVID-19, and much of the work to advance those initiatives predated the pandemic period. Yet, COVID-19 and the contemporaneous national reckoning with systemic oppression provided opportunities to instigate and sustain change.

This article describes how COVID-19 health disparities relate to the social determinants of health and reviews the importance of a diverse nursing workforce prepared to advance an antiracist framework for social justice. Throughout the article, we connect the past and present recommendations of the National Academy of Medicine (formerly the Institute of Medicine) about the "Future of Nursing" (FON) to contemporary antiracist and antioppressive frameworks. We then highlight practical strategies that exemplify the efforts of the Pennsylvania Action Coalition (PA-AC) to implement the recommendations of the FON reports through (1) mentoring nurses from underrepresented backgrounds, (2) amplifying diverse nursing voices, and (3) leveraging the power of coalitions. In highlighting the interwoven impact of COVID-19 and dramatic social change from 2020 to 2022, the article strives to inspire readers to move beyond the acute crisis of COVID-19 to the broader lens of sustained social justice in health care.

HISTORY

The Future of Nursing: Leading Change, Advancing Health (2010) created a blueprint for improving health care through targeted strategies that leverage the potential of the nursing workforce.[1] Broadly summarized, the recommendations included advancing nursing education, increasing leadership roles for nurses, removing barriers to nursing practice, and improving access to workforce data. Threaded throughout the report was the need for a diverse nursing workforce. When the Future of Nursing: Campaign for Action, assumed the role of implementing the recommendations of the FON report; they established "promoting diversity" as one of the pillars.[2]

In 2012, the PA-AC became one of 51 state action coalitions, and like the national campaign, embraced the recommendations related to diversity as core priorities around which to organize. Under the original leadership of Dr Dawndra Jones and Dr Rita K. Adeniran, the Nurse Diversity Council of the PA-AC (NDC) welcomed nurses and nurse advocates from across PA who saw the need for the state's nursing workforce to reflect the diverse populations it serves. The NDC set out to enhance nurses' knowledge, attitudes, and skills regarding diversity, promote inclusion in the nursing workforce, and foster culturally competent care. NDC stakeholders convened to define diversity "as all the ways in which we are similar and/or different… encompassing any dimension of human differences or similarities, including but not limited to cultural, cognitive, and social variables that differentiate groups of people from one another."[3]

Members of the NDC represent diverse backgrounds throughout Pennsylvania from a variety of health and health care settings. Members share their expertise to establish short- and long-term goals to promote a diverse and culturally competent nursing workforce. Since its founding, NDC members have met at least every other month via conference call for one hour to share progress on their action plans. The NDC has also created subcommittees as needed to execute targeted projects, such as conference planning.

Early NDC projects included short videos highlighting nurses from traditionally un-derrepresented backgrounds. In Video 1, nurses answered the question: "When did you know you wanted to become a nurse?" The NDC also supported a survey of Pennsylvania nurses related to cultural competency, which demonstrated a desire among nurses to be more culturally competent.[4,5]

Across the nation, the recommendations of the 2010 FON report sought to bolster the foundation of nursing to address what was already described as a troubled health care environment stemming from an aging population, fragmented system, uncontained costs, and questionable quality of care. The report could not have predicted COVID-19, but it could have more deeply addressed the profound impact that systemic racism has on health care and the social determinants of health. Future reports took on these issues directly.

The National Academy of Medicine continued its work to support the next decade of nursing, producing *Assessing Progress on the Institute of Medicine Report The Future of Nursing* in 2015[6] and began research for the FON 2020 in 2018. Meanwhile, national and international organizations strategized to take on the health care priorities of the next decade. The World Health Organization identified the year 2020 as the "International Year of the Nurse and Midwife."[7] Federal initiatives like Healthy People were likewise updating their strategies for the decade ahead.[8]

Ultimately, 2020 brought with it more than our health care and social institutions anticipated.

CONTEXT

The COVID-19 pandemic impacted every facet of life in 2020, and the foundation of nursing experienced unprecedented pressure, highlighting every crack along the way. US society entered another transformative period in 2020 with the murders of George Floyd, Breonna Taylor, Ahmaud Arbury, Tony McDade, and too many more.[9–11] COVID-19 further revealed the impact of systemic racism on the health and well-being of communities as the virus infected and killed black Americans at disproportionate rates from the beginning. Comprehending the full impact of COVID-19 requires understanding the "Color of COVID-19."[12] The pandemic period cannot be fully appreciated outside the context of America's centuries overdue reckoning with racism. **Box 1** includes the definitions of racism adopted in the FON report.

The COVID-19 pandemic dramatically exposed the ways people of color experience disparities in health care and inequities related to social determinants of health. Dr Camara Phyllis Jones, past president of the American Public Health Association, underscores that historical factors of systematic oppression led to disparate outcomes from COVID-19.[16,17] In an interview with Claudia Wallis with the *Scientific American*, Jones outlines how racism led to an increased disease burden of COVID-19:

1. People of color are less protected from and more exposed to the virus because they are more likely to live in disinvested communities that have less healthful options and poorer environmental factors such as air quality.
2. People of color are less likely to have access to high-quality health care; this led to a decreased ability to access testing and vaccines, and more broadly, receive the best care once in the hospital. In addition, people of color are more likely to experience individual and systemic discrimination once in the care of a health care provider.
3. People of color are more likely to hold frontline jobs that were classified as essential work and undervalued in terms of pay, including home health aides, postal workers, warehouse workers, meat packers, and hospital orderlies.

Box 1
Definitions of racism adopted in the future of nursing report[13–16]

Racism: An organized social system in which the dominant racial group, based on an ideology of inferiority, categorizes and ranks people into social groups called "races" and uses its power to devalue disempower, and differentially allocate valued societal resources and opportunities to groups defined as inferior.[13]

Racism is a structural inequity that negatively impacts health and health equity.[16]

Williams and colleagues[13,16] describe 3 interrelated forms of racism: structural racism, cultural racism, and discrimination.

Structural racism: Racism that is embedded in laws, policies, and institutions and provides advantages to the dominant racial group while oppressing, disadvantaging, or neglecting other racial groups. Structural racism can be seen in residential segregation, the criminal justice system, the public education system, and immigration policy. Williams and colleagues[13,16] identify structural racism as the most important way in which racism impacts health.

Cultural racism: The instillation of the ideology of inferiority in the values, language, imagery, symbols, and unstated assumptions of the larger society. Through cultural racism, people absorb and internalize negative stereotypes and beliefs about race, which can both create and support structural and individual racism and create implicit biases.[13,16]

Discrimination: It occurs when people or institutions treat racial groups differently, with or without intent, and this difference results in inequitable access to opportunities and resources.[13,16]

Intersectionality: Recognizes the complex factors contributing to health inequities by stressing the importance of the intersection of multiple interdependent social determinants that shape the health and well-being of individuals and communities. More specifically, the theoretical framework considers the intersection of these social determinants at the "micro level of individual experience to reflect multiple interlocking systems of privilege and oppression at the macro, social-structural level."[15]

The intersection of such social determinants as race, gender, and socioeconomic status is multiplicative rather than additive with respect to health outcomes.[14] Although there is a wealth of literature on social determinants of health, less literature is available on the intersection of social determinants and its impact on health outcomes. A full understanding of intersectionality will allow nurses to take a more holistic approach that considers the intersection of multiple interdependent social determinants that impact the health and well-being of individuals and communities.[16]

---

4. People of color are more vulnerable to disease because they are overrepresented in prisons and jails and immigration detention centers and are more likely to suffer from housing insecurity. These factors resulted in an increased likelihood of living in densely populated areas and/or areas that have poorer access to clean water.
5. People of color are less protected because their lives are less valued by cultural norms.
6. People of color are more likely to experience worse outcomes or die as a result of COVID-19 because they are more burdened with chronic diseases such as hypertension.[18–20] This increased burden is due to their increased likelihood of living in places with sparser access to tools that enable people to live healthier lives as a result of residential segregation.

Like the general population, nurses of color disproportionately suffered the impacts of COVID-19. Approximately 32% of health care worker deaths were among nurses **(Fig. 1)**,[21] and perhaps the most striking example of COVID-19's disparate impact was seen among Filipino nurses.[22]

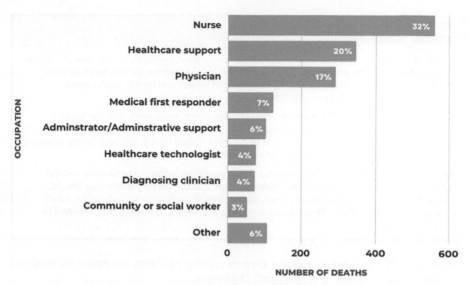

Fig. 1. Number of US health care worker deaths during first year of pandemic.[21]

Percentages represent number of healthcare worker deaths from a sample size of 1,734 people

The long-awaited *The Future of Nursing 2020-2030: Charting a Path to Achieve Health Equity* was published in May 2021 and referenced the research aforementioned alongside decades of research on racial disparities and social determinants of health. Beyond the existing pressures on the health care system explained in the original report, the new report was published as institutions were stretched to their limits managing an unrelenting public health crisis and as the nation was grappling with its legacy of racism and other systems of oppression. Among the 54 recommendations were changes needed to prevent the crises observed in 2020 and to build capacity to withstand future crises. **Boxes 2–5** include the recommendations most directly reflecting this context.

The recommendations of *the Future of Nursing 2020-2030* report solidified the path forward for Action Coalitions already working to cultivate a diverse nursing workforce. The report accurately reflected the priorities of the moment and bolstered the foundation laid by the PA-AC and its NDC since 2012.

PROMISING PRACTICES

The PA-AC has implemented several promising practices to advance workforce diversity and foster an environment of belonging among nurses from all backgrounds. This section focuses on 3 overlapping initiatives that illustrate these approaches: (1) mentoring future nurses from traditionally underrepresented backgrounds, (2) amplifying diverse nursing voices, and (3) leveraging the power of coalitions.

Pennsylvania Action Coalition Cohort of Exchanged Learning Mentorship Program

Creating a health care system that empowers everyone to live their healthiest lives requires the nursing workforce to be reflective of the population that it serves.[16] Diversifying the nursing pipeline entails more than recruiting and admitting a diverse student body. It is critical to build an inclusive environment where all students receive individualized support and are encouraged to thrive academically and professionally. During

---

Box 2
FON 2020 recommendations[16]

Recommendation 2: By 2023, state and federal government agencies, health care and public organizations, payers, and foundations should initiate substantive actions to enable the nursing workforce to address social determinants of health and health equity more comprehensively, regardless of practice setting.

Recommendation 3: By 2021, nursing education programs, employers, nursing leaders, licensing boards, and nursing organizations should initiate the implementation of structures, system, and evidence-based interventions to promote nurses' health and well-being, especially as they take on new roles to advance health equity

Recommendation 8: To enable nurses to address inequities within communities, federal agencies and other key stakeholders within and outside the nursing profession should strengthen and protect the nursing workforce during the response to such public health emergencies as the COVID-19 pandemic and natural disasters, including those related to climate change.

---

the pandemic, the need to support diverse nursing students increased as students navigated new personal and academic challenges.

In 2020, the NDC of the PA-AC and Lincoln University of Pennsylvania (Lincoln University) partnered to start the PA-AC Cohort of Exchanged Learning (PA-ACCEL). The objective of the program is to bolster nursing students' capacity to be successful in nursing school and in their transition to professional nursing practice. Through qualitative and quantitative feedback, the program has demonstrated a positive impact with regard to the students' and mentors' satisfaction. Since its inception, the PA-ACCEL program has been designed to be both sustainable with regard to the institution that it is serving and replicable to expand its reach to more students. The goal of the partnership between the PA-AC and Lincoln University was to provide comprehensive resources and programmatic support, recruit mentors, create evaluation tools, and maintain communications between Lincoln, the students, and the mentors. The PA-AC built a dedicated committee of PA-AC staff and partners to execute these tasks with Lincoln and to develop meaningful experiences for the students and mentors.

Box 3
Responses from student-mentees in the 2020 to 2021 and 2021 to 2022 cohort about what they learned about themselves so far

"I have learned to reach out to people in my career path"

"I have learned that I am open to learning about the different routes I can take with a nursing degree"

"...that there is nothing I cannot conquer"

"I am resilient, strong minded, and more capable than I believe myself to be"

I have learned..."To be myself and to advocate for yourself"

"... I'm stronger and know more than I think"

"I am very capable of achieving all my goals, and that setting goals has made life easier and more organized"

"I am a strong interviewer and planner"

Responses collected from the 2020-2021 and 2021-2022 PA-ACCEL Student-Mentee Program Evaluations.

> **Box 4**
> **Responses from student-mentees in the 2020 to 2021 and 2021 to 2022 cohort about how the coronavirus disease 2019 pandemic impacted them as a student**
>
> "I struggled mentally to keep going and trying to tell myself that i got this. I was very discouraged but also empowered. It just was difficult finding a balance"
>
> "Poor learning and communication with faculty and classroom settings"
>
> "I have been struggling with keeping up with everything and feeling motivated"
>
> "It impacted me by making me do a lot of things virtual and I feel Like I lost a lot of resources."
>
> "Not being to work at first to pay bills."
>
> "Covid-19 made things lot harder to manage me as a student"
>
> Responses collected from the 2020-2021 and 2021-2022 PA-ACCEL Student-Mentee Program Evaluations.

The PA-ACCEL addresses structural inequities in our health care system by equipping nurses from underrepresented backgrounds with more tools to pursue their educational goals and to be the health care leaders that they are fully capable of becoming. Lincoln University, the nation's first degree-granting Historically Black College and University (HBCU), reports that 85% of their students are black or African American,[23] whereas most nursing students across the country are white. In 2020, almost 81% of RNs reported being white.[24] Studies have shown that common barriers to the success for minority nursing students have included a lack of financial support; inadequate emotional, moral, and technical support; insufficient academic advising and program mentoring; and inadequate professional socialization.[25] The PA-ACCEL program components outlined below respond to these barriers, addressing the social determinant of health of educational attainment for the students who participate and the transformation of access to care and services for those who will benefit from their successful career as professional nurses.

The PA-ACCEL matches students with mentors recruited from the PA-AC's NDC. Students select their preferred mentors, according to their interests and desired career paths. The Mentor Biography Lookbook created for this past year's cohort includes the volunteer mentors' passions and professional roles. Students ranked their

> **Box 5**
> **Continuing the conversation about racism and coronavirus disease 2019 with Dr Deborah Washington[30]**
>
> "What nurses are doing, minority nurses, Black nurses are doing is to respond to the outreach of: This is what I need. Can you help us? Your voice carries weight. Can you help us to think about whether or not what we're asking for is feasible? How does the system operate?"
>
> "That the most powerful action we've taken in terms of how to message to a community within its cultural values. I can address vaccine hesitancy as a nurse, as a Black nurse, by tapping into the cultural values of Black people around the need to protect family and family relationships"
>
> "Nursing as a communicator, as a relational discipline, there's nothing better."
>
> "The most practical thing we can do these days is number one, to stop treating health disparities and inequities as sort of a crisis intervention"
>
> Additional quotes from Dr. Deborah Washington in "At the Core of Care" podcast episode, "Vaccine Hesitancy: Is Healthcare Listening?"

top 3 mentor choices according to this book. In the first cohort we received overwhelming interest in being a mentor, and many of the mentors indicated that they would be interested in serving as a mentor to an additional student. In the second cohort, the program expanded to both the junior and senior classes, because the program committee felt that the juniors might be able to receive enhanced benefits from their participation in the program. The mentor-mentee relationship is designed to continue into the students' senior year. We also received feedback that due to competing priorities of impending graduation and NCLEX preparation, the junior class would have more capacity than the senior class to be active in professional development opportunities.

Students and mentors receive individualized training, resources, and an outline of expectations for the year. Information is shared through separate meetings to introduce the program staff, facilitate a networking activity, walk through the compilation of tools, and answer any questions. At this point, we also review the comprehensive PA-ACCEL Toolkit, which details the program's purpose and expectations, tips for navigating the mentor and mentee relationship, resources specific to both students and mentors, and areas for further exploration.[26] Mentors sign commitment letters, where they agree to attend the trainings, meet with their mentee at least once a month for the entirety of one calendar year, and complete initial, midyear, and end-of-year evaluations. We ask for honest communication and feedback, outreach to the program committee with any issues, and their enthusiasm and willingness to teach and to learn. Students also sign agreement letters where they acknowledge their participation and program expectations.

The PA-ACCEL includes a robust evaluation process that consists of informal "check-in" surveys and a more formal mid-year and end-of-year evaluation questionnaire. The questions reflect the mentors' and mentees' experiences and goals. Responses from the end-of-year survey from the 2020-2021 cohort showed that 89% of students found the program to be helpful (this increased to 93% for the second cohort) and 75% of students reported that their mentor was a good match and plan to keep in touch after the program concludes. In addition, most students (93%) reported that using the PA-ACCEL Toolkit and other resources was helpful. Most impressively, 100% of students maintained a grade point average of 3.6 or higher in their last semester, and 100% of students from both cohorts are on track with their postgraduation goals. Examples of the students' goals include passing their NCLEX examination, pursuing higher education with plans to become a trauma nurse or nurse practitioner, entering the Air Force Nursing Transition Program, working in an intensive care unit, and working in a maternal-infant care unit. Furthermore, we received feedback to improve the infrastructure for the next cohort, including increasing communications between the cohort and the program committee and providing test-taking resources and tutoring for the NCLEX examination.

The students shared the comments listed in **Box 3** in response to the question asking what they had learned about themselves.

The PA-ACCEL program committee, including the PA-AC staff, Monica Harmon, Dr Vilma Davis (Director and Chair/Assistant Professor of the Nursing Department at Lincoln University), Dr Adriana Perez, Melanie Mariano, and Chavon Crampton, has navigated many hurdles in building a successful program. The team has met regularly since before the COVID-19 pandemic and remained connected to shift and reimagine the program's infrastructure to adapt to the pandemic environment. Frequent communication among all program partners to respond to students' concerns allowed the PA-ACCEL to succeed in its original goals despite difficulties presented by the pandemic. The team meets frequently to strategize in a collaborative, transparent environment.

One programmatic challenge was that, due to a variety of circumstances, not all students were able to fully engage at the level originally planned. Many students had competing priorities in their professional and personal lives. Although the program committee aimed to provide as much support as possible, remain available to students, and plan activities that were in tune with the students' interests and needs, ultimately the students need to decide to engage with the program on their own. **Box 4** describes challenges specific to the COVID-19 pandemic.

As part of the 2021-2022 Cohort, the PA-ACCEL included more leadership engagements for the students to expose them to public health advocacy in action and inspire a lifelong pursuit of health equity and justice. The opportunities were selected to showcase a variety of nursing pathways that students could explore in their careers and to provide tools for their professional growth. On February 3, 2022, the team traveled with 5 students to attend the National Black Nurses Day on Capitol Hill led by the National Black Nurses' Association, Inc (NBNA). The students had the opportunity to hear from esteemed nurse leaders and policy experts. Those who attended expressed that they had a rewarding experience and that they would recommend that their peers attend in future years. The PA-ACCEL also covered memberships to NBNA for each attending student, and will sponsor students to participate in the NBNA National Conference in Chicago from July 26 to 31, 2022. Another highlight from the year was the PA-ACCEL Professional Development Day, planned with support from the NDC. On April 6, 2022, the PA-AC hosted several panel presentations with the goal of increasing nursing students' confidence in their professional development and readiness to succeed in their transition to the nursing profession.

To broaden future participation in the program's activities, the PA-ACCEL provided additional networking opportunities and communications for the students. The program now includes more regular check-ins between students and mentors and monthly "office hours" sessions for mentors and mentees to connect with the program committee. The program hosted more regular "sharing out" of resources and other tools received from the broader PA-AC network. Crucially, despite the obstacles presented by the pandemic, the PA-ACCEL has cultivated and maintained a committed team that will help to ensure the program's sustainability and continued success. With a diversity of partnerships, including PA-AC staff, Lincoln University leadership, the PA-AC Advisory Board, and the NDC, the program is equipped to begin next year poised to make an even greater impact.

At the Core of Care Podcast: Amplifying Diverse Nursing Voices

At the Core of Care (ACC) highlights the consumer experience of patients, families, and communities and the creative efforts of nurses and other partners to better meet their health and health care needs through diversity, leadership, and practice innovation. The series received seed funding from the *Future of Nursing*: *Campaign for Action* Innovations Fund and is produced in partnership with Kouvenda Media, a social change multimedia production company.

Podcasting itself is emerging as a learning modality with the potential to reach diverse audiences and highlight a wide variety of voices. A wealth of podcasts focused on nursing have emerged in the last several years, including nurse-created independent podcasts, supplements to nursing journals and other publications, academic-based perspectives, and well-recognized institutional podcasts. Casting a wider net across health care, the Health Podcast Network "is a collection of over 8,000 podcast episodes that feature tough topics in health and care with empathy, expertise, and a commitment to excellence."[27] The podcasts each have a unique voice and together offer multifaceted insights into nursing and health care.

As a PA-AC initiative, ACC focuses primarily on highlighting diverse perspectives meeting special health care needs. When COVID-19 hit, podcast content naturally shifted to capture perspectives from the field. Highlighted in the following discussion are episodes that captured the seismic shifts related to diversity and COVID-19 through *At the Core of Care*.

2020: being heard

In "Social Justice in Nursing," Andre' Bennett, a graduate from Lincoln University, shares his outlook on what is happening in our country, the need for social justice, and how that relates to his interest in mental health nursing. The discussion highlights the intersection of contemporary events, the pandemic, and nursing institutions as presented through individual experience. "One of the nurse's main things and main objectives is to be an advocate for our patients. We are the buffer between our patients and sickness. And I think if we use that same drive that we have for our patients, we can make meaningful change not only with COVID but with the way the whole country is dealing with this whole racism piece. Audio 1"[28]

Similar to the Bennet interview, "Nursing Student Perspective on COVID-19" again highlighted the ways in which navigating the pandemic was shaped by one nurse's background. In this episode, we spoke with Ana Pichardo, a recent BSN graduate from LaSalle University and a full-time certified Spanish-speaking medical interpreter at Temple University Hospital in North Philadelphia. When her grandfather contracted the virus in another state, Pichardo functioned as her family's medical interpreter "not only with the language [because] most of my family doesn't speak English, but I also had to help them with the medical lingo."[29] She described the challenges of completing her nursing education while also watching her grandfather pass away on Zoom. However, she also described how the nurses who treated her grandfather helped her feel "part of the team" and solidified her decision to finish her degree to "become a nurse, so I can also be a support system for other families now dealing with this, because most likely with this pandemic, I will probably end up working with COVID patients. Audio 2"[29]

Both Bennett and Pichardo describe the importance of platforming diverse voices. Bennet said, "And I mean, as a African American male living now, hey, it's a tossup, whether you return home or not. *It's really important to be able to speak*."[28] Pichardo echoes the sentiment from a different perspective, with her experience helping her mother navigate the health care environment after coming from the Dominican Republic and not understanding English well. "And that's what first sparked my interest in medicine, to see my mom go through like all that hardship. *That bridge between not knowing the language and not being heard*."[28]

2021: "is health care listening"

When vaccines became available in late 2020, the discourse on diversity shifted to how to cultivate confidence in the vaccine among communities that have been mistreated by medical institutions for centuries. Through funding from the Centers for Disease Control and Prevention, *At the Core of Care* specifically addressed these issues across the country in early 2021.

Dr Deborah Washington, Director of Diversity for Nursing & Patient Care Services at Massachusetts General Hospital, directly confronted the issue of race and COVID-19 in "Vaccine Hesitancy: Is Healthcare Listening?" She describes the importance of having a more diverse nursing workforce and considering race in clinical trials—"the whole concept of racialized medicine Audio 3."[30] But what Washington most clearly notes is the strength of communities speaking out with their needs. "It's a change in the power dynamics of the community's voice in healthcare decision-making and healthcare strategizing."[30]

According to Washington, in Boston, the "system is listening" and, with the local community, rolled out strategies like community vaccination vans. And she noted that black nurses in particular have been important messengers not only to communities of color but also *from* communities of color. She notes that nurses with competing demands are not always making it to the community tables where strategizing and planning takes place. She is "trying to make that impression on communities of color here in Boston, that nursing as a discipline and nursing as a power broker absolutely has a place and influence in terms of helping you to reach your goals of access and care planning and disrupting things that need to change. *We do have a voice and you can trust us to do that work with you.*"[30] Additional quotes from the episode are available in **Box 5**.

In "Vaccine Confidence: Identifying Trusted Messengers," nurses spoke about reaching Asian and Arab-American communities in Michigan, with Philippine, black, and other diverse communities frequently echoing the same themes noted by Washington. Dr Meriam Caboral-Stevens, a researcher and faculty member at Eastern Michigan University in the School of Nursing and faculty at the university's Center for Health Disparities Innovations and Studies, described the importance of not only ensuring communities have access to technology and that their specific concerns are addressed but also the need for translated materials. She also described the importance of working within the religious culture of communities, like engaging the Imam when trying to connect with the Muslim community.

Opeyemi Ogunniyi, who works on a medical surgical unit in Houston, Texas, shared yet another perspective: "where I come from Nigeria, most people did not believe that COVID existed, they thought it was all a lie. Not until later last year to this year, when people were passing away and they found out that some of the symptoms were related to COVID because most of the symptoms of COVID, they believed there was malaria. So they'd never believed that it was COVID, they thought it was just like a made up term from the US."[31] Reglita Laput, the last nurse highlighted in this episode, is a community health nurse in Michigan (and president of the Philippine Nurses Association). Regardless of the setting, each nurse describes the essential roles that nurses can play. Ogunniyi says, "the community look up to us. In terms of what we put out there, *we're almost like, like a guide.* So that says a lot on the role of a nurse in the eyes of a patient."[31]

2022: looking ahead

Among the lessons reflected throughout the interviews, the need for nurses to not only listen but also speak out came through. As health care moves farther from the period of acute crisis, our speakers have increasingly called out the systems that still need to change. In "Cultivating Support, Resilience and Retention among Health Professions," Dr Paula Milone-Nuzzo discussed the continued need to reframe training and education for health professions. She talked about the need to "look internally at what aspects are inconsistent with an antiracism and anti-oppression framework"[32] from how case studies and assessments are taught to how faculty are supported. She describes a system that has been calling for the same improvements—better academic-practice partnership, pay that values the care that nurses provide, and allowing all health professions to practice to the top of their license. "And that's going to require sometimes changes in legislation, sometimes changes in statute, sometimes changes in accreditation standards. All of that is possible, because we are in a new area of healthcare."[32]

Nurse Diversity Council: Leveraging the Power of Coalitions

The pandemic exposed and exacerbated many problematic social realities, but it also elevated practices and approaches that foster resilience. The value of embracing diverse viewpoints and aligning multisector approaches was not new to the PA-AC during COVID-19, but the pandemic offered an opportunity to commit to it further.

Although some stakeholders pulled away into competing priorities, more partners deeply engaged in the coalition's work during the pandemic, sharing their unique perspectives and calling for joint action. At times when action felt like too much, simply connecting with colleagues in a different part of the state, from a different organization, often a different industry was an essential reminder that even folks shouldering tremendous responsibility still need a place to lean. In coalition work, and especially the work of collective impact initiatives, the importance of sharing measurable outcomes as a mechanism for aligning action stands out.[33] Although important, it is also possible that the less visible outcomes of coalition work are what kept people engaged during periods of professional and personal crisis.

As *The Future of Nursing 2020-2030: Charting a Path to Achieve Health Equity* was released, the PA-AC NDC felt that it was important to digest the report together and review the Council's mission and vision as it related to the new FON report. Although NDC members endured personal and professional burdens and traumas as the pandemic was surging, the group also knew that the calls in the report as they related to addressing health disparities were critical. The NDC listened to stakeholders in providing the space for dialogue and action, with a consensus to revisit its original charter in the new FON report's wake. The NDC recognized the danger in delaying these conversations for a time that was not a crisis because it is inherently in a crisis when disparities are underscored.

The NDC worked for months to bolster its charter, ultimately expanding to include the following:

> The NDC of the PA-AC is a volunteer council dedicated to promoting diversity and cultural humility in nursing to increase access and quality of care.
> The NDC aims to:
> - Enhance nurses' knowledge, attitudes, and skills regarding diversity, equity, and social determinants of health;
> - Work to promote equity, health equity, and health care equity;
> - Promote inclusion in the nursing workforce;
> - Foster culturally humble care across practice settings and levels;
> - Increase the diversity of the nursing workforce across academic pipelines; and
> - Educate the nursing workforce on structural racism, antiracist practices, and social and emotional justice.

Each meeting of the NDC begins with the verbal affirmation of each person present to make the meeting a "Gracious Space."[34] Gracious Space is a spirit and setting that invites the stranger and embraces learning in public.[35] "To invite the stranger" is defined as being open to diverse perspectives to gain clarity. "Learning in public" is defined as truly listening to new thoughts or conflicting ideas, with openness to changing one's mind. The power of a coalition to impact change resonates, because no one person, organization, industry, discipline, state, culture, race, or perspective can alone achieve the transformation required of society. Creating a Gracious Space in a coalition amplifies its power.

Action Coalitions are designed to foster cross-sector collaborations as they work to advance a culture of health equity. Best practices in coalition building increasingly frame activities in terms of leadership building and systems change. The *Future of Nursing*: *Campaign for Action*'s Health Equity Toolkit provides additional guidance for coalitions taking an upstream approach to public health and equity.[36]

Capturing the power of coalitions as a measurable outcome might look like the call for mentors for PA-ACCEL, which produced 4 times more mentors than mentees (15 students, 57 interested mentors). It might also look like the Cultural Competence Education and Awareness Survey that reached 1246 registered nurses in Pennsylvania through distribution among PA-AC networks.[4] The NDC has harnessed its collective power to produce 3 statewide conferences on diversity, the most recent in 2021 pivoting to entirely virtual content (**Fig. 2**). **Fig. 2** showcases the impact of the "Pennsylvania's Healthcare Mosaic" (Mosaic) conferences, sharing quantitative and qualitative feedback.

The Mosaic conference, cohosted by the PA-AC's NDC, is a biannual conference that gathers health and social service providers to share ideas surrounding health equity, diversity, inclusivity, culturally humble care, and cultural humility. Although each year has its own theme, the Mosaic conference seeks to open dialogue about health disparities, often created by the social determinants of health, and how they affect population health and the health care environment.

In 2016, the NDC hosted its first conference at the Robert Morris University School of Nursing and Health Sciences entitled "Pennsylvania's Healthcare Mosaic: Building a Culture of Health Equity." The next conference Pennsylvania's Healthcare Mosaic 2018 included partnering with the Drexel University College of Nursing and Health Professions with the theme of "Achieving Excellence in Care for All." Keynoting the conference was former Deputy Surgeon General Rear Admiral Sylvia Trent-Adams, PhD, RN, FAAN. Trent-Adams discussed the need to bridge gaps and build a Culture of Health while providing insight from her role advising operations of the US Public Health Service Commissioned Corps. "Culture is complex," Trent-Adams said. "This is hard work, but it's worth it."

In response to public health best practices, the NDC pivoted to host a virtual conference from March 1 to 5, 2021. In partnership with the Penn State College of Nursing, the "Pennsylvania's Healthcare Mosaic: Advocacy & Equity in Action" Virtual Conference brought together health care experts to (1) identify culturally competent care practices among academic, clinical, community, and other stakeholders; (2) discuss impact of health policy and advocacy on health, health care delivery, and outcomes; (3) examine current policy and evidence-based practices in addressing social determinants of health, health disparities, and health equity; and (4) analyze sources of explicit and implicit bias and how they affect patient care, community health, and health care policy. Like the earlier events, the conference galvanized advocates for health equity around nursing workforce strategies, not deterred by COVID-19 but poised to affect change.

SUMMARY

The COVID-19 pandemic offers lessons on diversity that unfortunately continue to be learned and learned again. The impact of the virus varied across minority populations as the same groups that suffer under systems of oppression were likewise more vulnerable to COVID-19. Moreover, the pandemic bolstered the role of the nurse as communicator and trusted advocate, emphasizing the value of a diverse nursing workforce to meet the needs of a diverse population. Efforts to increase nursing workforce diversity continue, and the context of the pandemic period along with calls for social change provides opportunities to amplify and scale existing strategies. Meanwhile,

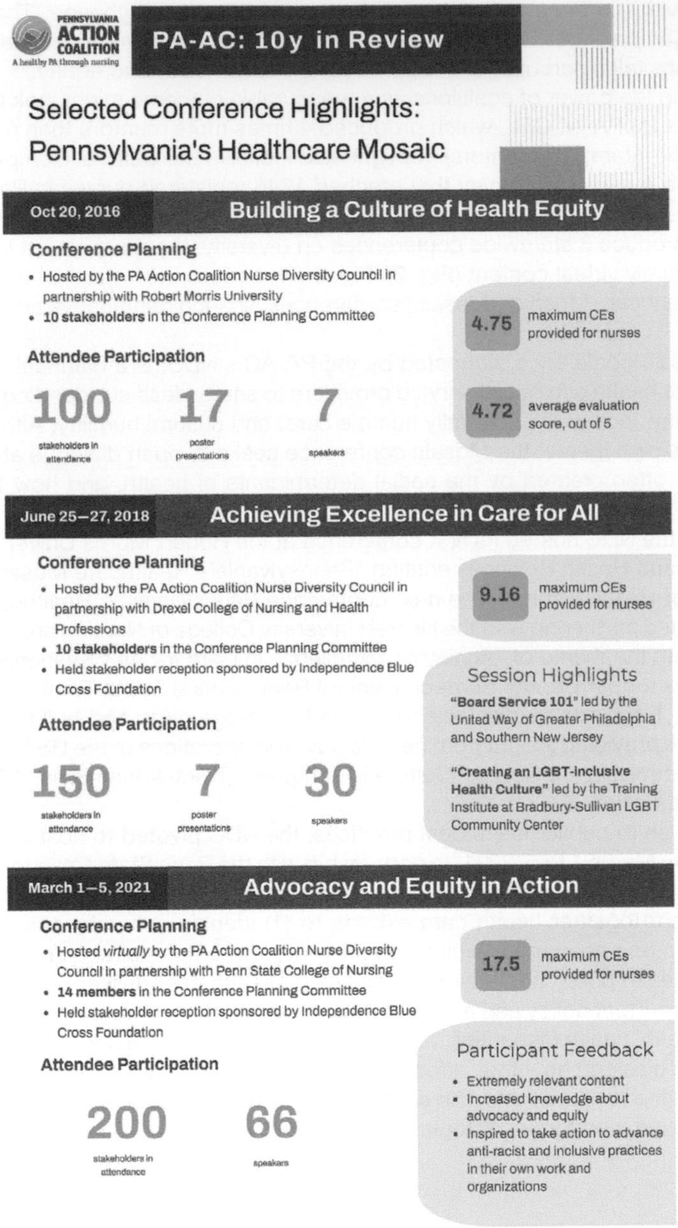

Fig. 2. Pennsylvania Action Coalition: 10 years in review—selected conference highlights: Pennsylvania's Healthcare Mosaic.[37]

preparing existing and future nurses to apply antiracist and antioppressive frameworks to their practice will build workforce capacity to address the unequal burden of social determinants of health. Ultimately, it will be the work of diverse stakeholders—the work of coalitions—that will apply the lessons learned during the COVID-19 pandemic to advance health equity.

CLINICS CARE POINTS

- Gracious Space creates a space for thoughtful dialogue and creative problem-solving.
- Nurses in all settings serve as communicators across individuals, families, and communities and the systems impacting them.
- Social injustice is not a short-term crisis; the lessons we have learned in the past several years need to transform health care for lasting change.
- Underrepresented nurses and communities need to be heard, which means health care needs to listen.
- Coalition work aligns diverse strengths that, when translated into action, produces substantial collective impact.

DISCLOSURE

The authors have nothing to disclose.

ACKNOWLEDGMENTS

Rita K. Adeniran, DRNP, RN, CMAC, NEA-BC, FNAP, FAAN. Dawndra Jones, DNP, RN, NEA-BC. Andre Bennet. Reglita Laput, MPHM, BSN, RN. Paula Milone-Nuzzo, PhD, RN, FHHC, FAAN. Opeyemi Ogunniyi, BSN, RN. MaryGrace Joyce, MS. Meriam Caboral-Stevens, PhD, RN. Wandia Mureithi, MPH. Vilma Davis, PNP, BC, PhD. Adriana Perez, PhD, CRNP, ANP-BC, FAAN, FGSA. Melanie Mariano, DNP, MSN, MPH, RN. Sharvette Philmon, MSN, RN, NEA-BC, CNE. Chavon Crampton, MSN, RNC-MNN, CLC, EFM-C. Sheldon D. Fields, PhD, RN, CRNP, FNP-BC, AACRN, FAANP, FNAP, FAAN. Roberta Waite, EdD, MSN, PMHCNS, ANEF, FAAN. Rear Admiral (retired) Sylvia Trent-Adams, PhD, RN, FAAN. Susan B. Hassmiller, RN, PhD, FAAN. Nurse Diversity Council. Kouvenda Media. PA-AC Advisory Board.

SUPPLEMENTARY DATA

Supplementary data related to this article can be found online at https://doi.org/10.1016/j.cnur.2022.10.003.

REFERENCES

1. Institute of Medicine. The future of nursing: leading change, advancing health. The National Academies Press; 2011. https://doi.org/10.17226/12956.
2. Campaign for Action. Issue: Increasing Diversity in Nursing. campaignforaction.org. https://campaignforaction.org/term-issue/increasing-diversity-in-nursing/. [Accessed 1 July 2022].
3. PA Action Coalition. Diversity. paactioncoalition.org. 2019. https://www.paactioncoalition.org/initiatives/diversity.html. [Accessed 1 July 2022].
4. Adeniran RJ, Jones D, Harmon MJ, et al. Checking the Pulse of Holistic and Culturally Competent Nursing Practice in Pennsylvania. Holist Nurs Pract 2020. https://doi.org/10.1097/HNP.0000000000000427.
5. The Pennsylvania Action Coalition. When Did You Know You Wanted to Be a Nurse? paactioncoalition.org. 2016. https://www.paactioncoalition.org/youtube-videos/item/457-when-did-you-know-you-wanted-to-be-a-nurse.html. [Accessed 1 July 2022].

6. National Academies of Sciences. Engineering, and medicine. Assessing progress on the Institute of medicine report the future of nursing. The National Academies Press; 2016. https://doi.org/10.17226/21838.

7. Executive Board designates 2020 as the "Year of the Nurse and Midwife". World Health Organization. 2019. https://www.who.int/news/item/30-01-2019-executive-board-designates-2020-as-the-year-of-the-nurse-and-midwife-. [Accessed 1 July 2022].

8. Office of Disease Prevention and Health Promotion. Healthy People 2030 Framework. health.gov. https://health.gov/healthypeople/about/healthy-people-2030-framework. [Accessed 1 July 2022].

9. Minkler M, Wakimoto P. Community organizing and community building for health and social equity. 4th edition. Rutgers University Press; 2021.

10. Zinzi BD, Feldman JM, Bassett MT. How structural racism works - racist policies as a root cause of US racial health inequities. N Engl J Med 2021;384:768–73.

11. Kendi IX. Our new postracial myth. The Atlantic. 2021. https://www.theatlantic.com/ideas/archive/2021/06/our-new-postracial-myth/619261/. [Accessed 1 July 2022].

12. Gawthrop E. The Color of Coronavirus: COVID-19 deaths by race and ethnicity in the U.S. apmresearchlab.org. 2022. https://www.apmresearchlab.org/covid/deaths-by-race#:~:text=Our%20ongoing%20Color%20of%20Coronavirus,deaths%20in%20the%20United%20States. [Accessed 1 July 2022].

13. Williams DR, Lawrence JA, Davis BA. Racism and health: Evidence and needed research. Annu Rev Public Health 2019;40:105–25.

14. Assari S. Social determinants of depression: The intersections of race, gender, and socioeconomic status. Brain Sci 2017;7(12). https://doi.org/10.3390/brainsci7120156.

15. Bowleg L. The problem with the phrase women and minorities: Intersectionality—an important theoretical framework for public health. Am J Public Health 2012;102(7):1267–73.

16. National Academies of Sciences. Engineering, and medicine. The future of nursing 2020-2030: charting a path to achieve health equity. The National Academies Press; 2021. p. 38.

17. Wallis C. Why racism, not race, is a risk factor for dying of COVID-19. Scientific American: Public Health. 2020. https://www.scientificamerican.com/article/why-racism-not-race-is-a-risk-factor-for-dying-of-covid-191/. [Accessed 1 July 2022].

18. Office of Minority Health, HHS. Diabetes and African Americans. minorityhealth.hhs.gov. 2021. https://minorityhealth.hhs.gov/omh/browse.aspx?lvl=4&lvlid=18. [Accessed 1 July 2022].

19. Office of Minority Health, HHS. Heart disease and African Americans. minorityhealth.hhs.gov. 2022. https://minorityhealth.hhs.gov/omh/browse.aspx?lvl=4&lvlid=19. [Accessed 1 July 2022].

20. Yancy CW. COVID-19 and African Americans. J Am Med Assoc 2020;323(19):1891–2.

21. The Guardian. Lost on the frontline. thegaurdian.com. 2021. https://www.theguardian.com/us-news/ng-interactive/2020/dec/22/lost-on-the-frontline-our-findings-to-date. [Accessed 1 July 2022].

22. Diaz D, Caboral-Stevens M. Health-promoting behavior and positive mental health of Filipino nurses in Michigan. J Nurs Pract Appl Rev Res 2021;11(1):39–42. Available at: https://www.emich.edu/chdis/documents/stevens/jnparr-2021.pdf. [Accessed 1 July 2022].

23. Lincoln University. Statistical overview. Lincoln University 2018-2019 Annual Report. 2019:16. https://www.lincoln.edu/_files/annual-reports/annual-report-2019.pdf. [Accessed 1 July 2022].

24. Richard A, Ruttinger C, Oliveira CM, et al. The 2020 National Nursing Workforce Survey. J Nurs Regul 2021;12(1):1–96.

25. Dorsey LE, Baker CM. Mentoring undergraduate nursing students assessing the state of the science. Nurse Educator 2004;29(6):260–5.

26. Harmon MJ, Perez A, Bird J, et al. PA-AC Cohort of Exchanged LEarning (PA-AC-CEL) 2021-2022 Cohort: Mentor-Mentee Toolkit. Pennsylvania Action Coalition. 2021. https://www.paactioncoalition.org/images/PA-ACCEL/2021-2022/PA-ACCEL_Mentee-Mentor_Toolkit_102021.pdf. [Accessed 1 July 2022].

27. Health Podcast Network. About. healthpodcastnetwork.com. https://healthpodcastnetwork.com/about/. [Accessed 1 July 2022].

28. PA Action Coalition, Social Justice in Nursing. At the Core of Care. 2020. https://www.paactioncoalition.org/about/podcast/scripts/item/579-social-justice-in-nursing.html. [Accessed 1 July 2022].

29. PA Action Coalition, Nursing Student Perspective of COVID-19. At the Core of Care. 2020. https://www.paactioncoalition.org/about/podcast/scripts/item/576-nursing-student-perspective-of-covid-19.html. [Accessed 1 July 2022].

30. PA Action Coalition, Vaccine Hesitancy: Is Healthcare Listening?. At the Core of Care. 2021. https://www.paactioncoalition.org/about/podcast/scripts/item/628-vaccine-hesitancy-is-healthcare-listening.html. [Accessed 1 July 2022].

31. PA Action Coalition, Vaccine Confidence: Identifying Trusted Messengers. At the Core of Care. 2021. https://www.paactioncoalition.org/about/podcast/scripts/item/637-vaccine-confidence-identifying-trusted-messengers.html. [Accessed 1 July 2022].

32. PA Action Coalition, Cultivating Support, Resilience and Retention for the Health Professions. At the Core of Care. 2022. https://www.paactioncoalition.org/about/podcast/scripts/item/685-cultivating-support-resilience-and-retention-for-the-health-professions.html. [Accessed 1 July 2022].

33. Kania John, Kramer Mark. Collective Impact. Stanford Social Innovation Rev 2011;9(1):36–41.

34. Nurse Diversity Council (NDC). Gracious Space. paactioncoalition.org. Available at: https://www.paactioncoalition.org/initiatives/diversity.html.

35. Hughes PM, Grace B. Gracious space: a practical guide for working better together. Seattle, Washington: The Center for Ethical Leadership; 2004 (See Available at: http://ethicalleadership.org. [Accessed 1 July 2022].

36. Ackerman-Barger K, Cooper J, Eddie R, et al. Building Coalitions To Promote Health Equity: A Toolkit for Action. Future of Nursing: Campaign for Action. 2022. https://campaignforaction.org/wp-content/uploads/2022/04/AARP_CCNA_HealthEquityToolkit_Revi_051122.pdf. [Accessed 1 July 2022].

37. Mureithi, W. PA-AC 10 Years in Review: Selected Conference Highlights: Pennsylvania's Healthcare Mosaic. Pennsylvania Action Coalition. Accessed June 27, 2022.

Instilling Confidence in the COVID-19 Vaccine

Kristine Gonnella, MPH[a],*, Deepa Mankikar, MPH[b,1]

KEYWORDS

- COVID-19 • Vaccine confidence • Social media • Social marketing • Nurses
- Trusted messengers

KEY POINTS

- The professional nursing community is active on social media and engages with social media content.
- Paid advertising was an effective strategy to promote vaccine confidence content and expand reach of the social media campaign.
- Nurses were more likely to reshare existing content from trusted organizations on their social feed.
- Consider offering trainings to social media campaign followers to increase their online presence and comfort in posting.

The Nurses Make Change Happen media campaign engaged audiences nationally to promote vaccine confidence and get vaccinated through leveraging nurses as micro-influencers. The campaign found success using a softer, nonconfrontational approach to messaging. Posts that used real nurses to encourage rather than demand the target audience to get vaccinated were more well received. Paid ads helped increase channel followers of National Nurse-Led Care Consortium (NNCC) and encouraged resharing of content. Targeted ads were a successful strategy based on cost-per-click (CPC) and the click-through rate (CTR).

BACKGROUND

On March 11, 2020, the World Health Organization declared coronavirus disease 2019 (COVID-19) a global pandemic. From March 2020 through April 2020, infection rates continued to surge around the world and subsequent hospitalizations increased. Despite global stay-at-home orders in place, nurses critical to mitigation of COVID-19, continued care provision.[1] Nurses played an essential role in COVID-19 response,

[a] Public Health Management Corporation, Philadelphia, PA, USA; [b] National Nurse-Led Care Consortium, Philadelphia, PA, USA
[1] Present address: 4601 Market Street, Philadelphia, PA 19139.
* Corresponding author. 1500 Market Street, Philadelphia, PA 19102.
E-mail address: kgonnella@phmc.org

Nurs Clin N Am 58 (2023) 77–85
https://doi.org/10.1016/j.cnur.2022.11.001
0029-6465/23/© 2022 Elsevier Inc. All rights reserved.

Table 1 Tracking Impact of Media Campaign	
Objective	**Metrics**
Objective 1: Generate vaccine confidence toolkit website traffic and downloads on a microsite	• Number of website clicks to NNCC (CPC) • Number of in-feed kit downloads (CPD)
Objective 2: Create engagement through shared content	• Social posts shared or originated from NNCC content (hashtag, tag tracking) • Engagements (likes, comments, shares)
Objective 3: Build awareness of NNCC in the professional nurse community to elevate the role of nurses *Objective 4:* Build COVID-19 vaccine awareness for consumers who are vaccine hesitant or in low vaccination areas/states	• Brand impressions, number of website clicks • Percent of the audience reached

The campaign tailored vaccine messaging to reach defined target professional and consumer audiences. NNCC worked to further defined audience segments, including nursing professionals, individuals in public health/community roles, vaccine-hesitant individuals, and parents. NNCC identified these audiences and the approximate reach across social media platforms through a combination of (1) selection criteria available through social media account management targeting age groups, industry, educational level, and geographic level and (2) Hashtags or Keywords on what individuals search or include in posts who fit these criteria. For example, NNCC could identify its target parent audience on Twitter by using keywords (suggested from Twitter) on what individuals search or include in posts who are talking about child vaccination, such as "fertility vaccines," "family vaccine," "children vaccinated," "pregnant vaccination," to name a few. Social media platforms vary in the extent to which audiences can be targeted. After segmenting the audience based on industry, demographics and age, NNCC further narrowed the list by overlaying data for states with under 50% vaccination rates and other key demographics.

The nurse-led vaccine confidence microinfluencer campaign was active across various social media channels including Facebook, Instagram, LinkedIn, and Twitter. The content was defined by 5 message types: addressing vaccine hesitancy, nurse advice, personal nurse story, resources, and promoting the social toolkit. Twenty-nine ads were created to support all audiences, with different channel versions. During the campaign, states that fell into the bottom five states with vaccine rates were included in the media buy. The campaign was expanded to the bottom seven states with additional funding. Overall, the campaign cost a total budget of US$75,000. As part of the campaign strategy, organic content was also created in addition to using paid ads. This included 93 campaign posts, which led to an increase in NNCC followers on Facebook and LinkedIn. Additionally, NNCC launched a new Instagram account during this process resulting in 95 total followers with 315 individuals viewing the NNCC Instagram page during the campaign period.

DISCUSSION

The "Nurses Make Change Happen" campaign, which ran in two parts between June 2021 – June 2022, resulted in over 10.8M impressions, 62.4K website clicks, and 17.6K site actions (views of toolkit or campaign landing page). The campaign included targeted messaging to the top seven U.S. states with low COVID-19 vaccine rates in

2022. The first part of NNCC's campaign, from June 2021 - September 2021, produced over 4.0M impressions and 10.3K website clicks. The second part of NNCC's campaign, from February 2022 - July 2022, resulted in over 6.7M impressions; 52.1K website clicks; 17.6K site actions (views of toolkit or campaign landing page); and 18 toolkit shares from the microsite (**Table 2**).

Table 2
Nurses Make Change Happen Campaign Impact

Campaign Timeframe	Impressions	Website Clicks	Site Actions	Toolkit Shares
Part 1 (June 2021 – September 2021)	4,025,345	10,299	N/A	N/A
Part 2 (February 2022 – July 2022)	6,781,801	52,180	17,690	18

The campaign reached 46% of the nurse professional community on Facebook, 6.6% on Twitter and 3.0% on LinkedIn. The campaign also reached 65% of the vaccine hesitant community on Twitter and 22% on Facebook. Sixty-four percent of the parents' audience was reached on Twitter and 4.6% on Facebook (**Table 3**).

Table 3
Nurses make change happen campaign reach

Social Media Platform	Campaign Reach	Audience Size	Audience Reached (%)
Facebook			
Nurse Professional Community	259,760	555,300	46.8%
Public Health Services	62,608	549,700	11.4%
Vaccine Hesitant Individuals	293,635	1,300,000	22.6%
Current and Hopeful Parents	156,787	3,400,000	4.6%
LinkedIn			
Nurse Professional Community	118,581	4,000,000	3.0%
Public Health Services	42,299	610,000	6.9%
Twitter			
Nurse Professional Community	616,549	9,300,000	6.6%
Public Health Services	139,656	214,700	65.0%
Vaccine Hesitant Individuals	97,572	150,200	65.0%
Current and Hopeful Parents	67,001	104,700	64.0%

Through back-end data of the social media accounts, NNCC learned more details on demographics of people who viewed particular content. For example, Women ages 25-34 interacted most with the nurse stories. Men of various ages were interested in the campaign's video content and nurse interviews more than still graphics and showed a heightened interest in messages that dispelled myths around fertility and COVID-19. The back-end data collected was used to further refine the approach to target our defined audience and adjust campaign content and format.

The cost per click (CPC) at US$1.43 was impressive, proving a cost-effective way to reach and engage with the identified audiences. In comparison, the average CPC for health and medical content is US $2.62.[21] The campaign goal was to drive site traffic. NNCC had a total of 52,180 website clicks with 21% going to the social media toolkit and 79% going to the campaign landing page. On the campaign landing page, a microsite linked to the main NNCC website, approximately 92% of total visitors came from paid media. The nurse story content had the highest CTR at 1.4%, compared with the next highest category, which were posts on nurse advice at 1.1%. This shows personalized content with real names and faces was driving higher clicks compared with other content shared. Of all the audiences, vaccine-hesitant individuals had the highest CTR at 1.1%, indicating the messages resonated and were clicked on to learn more. The vaccine-hesitant audience was highly active when being targeted on social media. The social media toolkit was designed to encourage content sharing by the nursing community. However, one shortfall NNCC observed is that although ads drove people to the microsite (6.9 K clicks; 3.7 K site views), there was minimal sharing of the social content (18 shares). Although nurses were not as likely to create their own content or share the toolkit, they were highly engaged in viewing and accessing the microsite. Nurses were also more likely to reshare existing NNCC published content on their own social media feeds, demonstrating paid ads can encourage content sharing when posted by a trusted source, in this case, a national nursing membership organization.

Leveraging professional expertise on social media to promote public health initiatives is an emerging area of opportunity. The COVID-19 pandemic demonstrated the opportunities and challenges with rapid dissemination of information and the complexity of ongoing vetting of trusted information and misinformation.[22] Establishing protocols and managing information dissemination among stakeholders may help minimize the spread of misinformation where inaccurate information becomes "fact." Establishing the need to create clear boundaries between personal and professional persona on social media is an area of further research.

Through the campaign, it was exciting to observe the nurse professional audience engage in social media content and content sharing; however, minimal sharing of the toolkit suggests nurses were not as comfortable creating their own content for social media or perhaps were hesitant to post it to their own personal social media accounts. To support nurses' ability to elevate their role as trusted health messengers and build their confidence in creating and maintaining an online presence, further training may be necessary. At the launch of NNCC's "Nurses Make Change Happen" Campaign, NNCC offered a Social Media and Media Training Workshop to promote nurses' skills and competencies on how to responsibly leverage and manage social media to share vaccine facts, address misinformation, serve as a vaccine ambassador, and navigate social media along with respect to the nursing code of ethics.

The nursing code of ethics, as developed by the American Nurses Association (ANA), is a guide for "carrying out nursing responsibilities in a manner consistent with quality in nursing care and the ethical obligations of the profession."[23] Trust is critical to the nurse, patient, and community relationship. Compromising this trusted relationship, even unintentionally, may damage the relationships developed among nurses and the communities they serve and the ongoing trust of the nursing profession. It is imperative that nurses always ensure that anything posted or published never undermines a patient treatment or privacy relationship with their communities.

With that in mind, the ANA created a set of principles to guide nurses when using social media, allowing nurses to get the best out of it while safeguarding themselves, the profession, and their patients. Many of the principles are common sense and should be standard practice for anyone experienced in using social media responsibly.

However, as the nursing profession continues to establish a professional presence on social media and promotes the use of social media as a tool to advance public health initiatives, the principles outlined by ANA below provide a helpful guide to responsibly engage with social channels.

1. Nurses must not transmit or place online individually identifiable patient information.
2. Nurses must observe ethically prescribed professional patient–nurse boundaries.
3. Nurses should understand that patients, colleagues, organizations, and employers may view postings.
4. Nurses should take advantage of privacy settings and seek to separate personal and professional information online.
5. Nurses should bring content that could harm a patient's privacy, rights, or welfare to the attention of appropriate authorities.
6. Nurses should participate in developing organizational policies governing online conduct.[24]

Before the COVID-19 pandemic, the image of nurses in the media was minimal and when present often rife with stereotypes.[8,9] Social media presents an opportunity for nurses to advance their image and harness media to reframe and promote the nursing profession, advance public health initiatives and indirectly promote improved health outcomes. The need to build confidence in the COVID-19 vaccines was a chance for nurses to be empowered and leverage their role as trusted messengers. As evidenced by the COVID-19 pandemic, the nursing code of ethics must be strictly adhered to so as not to compromise the integrity of the profession. Thus, more trainings are necessary to support health professionals navigate how to responsibly create and maintain an online presence.

SUMMARY

Leveraging nurses as micro-influencers, the "Nurses Make Change Happen" campaign engaged audiences nationally to promote vaccine confidence and encourage vaccine uptake. The campaign found success using a softer, nonconfrontational approach to messaging, for example, "talk to a nurse if you are hesitant" instead of "get your vaccine today." Posts that used real nurses to encourage rather than demand the target audience to get vaccinated were more well received. Paid ads helped increase NNCC's channel followers and encouraged resharing of content. Targeted ads were a successful strategy based on CPC and the CTR.

Through the campaign, we observed that the larger professional nursing community is active on social media and engages with content, and advertising was a great tactic to even promote additional content (eg, nurse trainings) and engagement with NNCC. Involving nurses from our VCAC proved to be an effective strategy for content and message development that was personal and representative of the audiences to be reached. Posts featuring nurses familiar with vaccine confidence and community engagement had the most success. Individuals are not as likely to personalize and share content, similar to the vaccine toolkit, but more likely to reshare existing content from trusted organizations on their social feed. This is a potential area to improve on in future campaigns by offering trainings to campaign followers to increase their online presence and comfort in posting.

Although we had organic traffic engage with our content, paid media had the most impact in expanding our reach and affecting our metrics. Momentum on Instagram was successful, and we anticipate continuing to publish content there to build a following. Directionally, the paid campaign helped to increase channel followers that will now see our organic content, which is an added earned benefit.

Nurses are recognized as trusted messengers, yet there is an absence of nurse presence in media. The COVID-19 pandemic provided an opportunity to encourage vaccine confidence and increaseuptake through leveraging the trusted voices of nurses through social media. The "Nurses Make Change Happen" social media campaign highlighted an emerging opportunity for nurses to create and promote public policy, have more visibility in media, and maximize their role as trusted messengers in health care.

CLINICS CARE POINTS

- There is an absence of positive nurse images in media.
- The absence of positive images and perpetuated stereotypes has negative consequences on the recruitment and retention of nurses as well as indirectly patient care.
- The COVID-19 pandemic highlighted the critical need of nurses on the front lines of health care.
- Social media was critical to information dissemination, both misinformation and trusted information.
- The racial, ethnic, and professional diversity of nurses as trusted messengers must be represented in media to combat the stereotypical image of the nursing profession.
- Paid media advertising, segmenting audiences, and targeted messaging are effective ways to promote vaccine confidence.

DISCLOSURE

The authors have nothing to disclose.

FUNDING

This project was funded in part by a cooperative agreement with the Centers for Disease Control and Prevention (grant number NU50CK000580). The Centers for Disease Control and Prevention is an agency within the Department of Health and Human Services (HHS). The contents of this resource center do not necessarily represent the policy of CDC or HHS and should not be considered an endorsement by the Federal Government.

REFERENCES

1. Fawaz M, Anshasi H, Samaha A. Nurses at the front line of COVID-19: roles, responsibilities, risks, and rights. Am J Trop Med Hyg 2020;103(4):1341–2.
2. The impact of COVID-19 on the nursing workforce: a national overview. Online J Issues Nurs 2021;26(2):N.PAG.
3. Salmond SW, Echevarria M. Healthcare transformation and changing roles for nursing. Orthop Nurs 2017;36(1):12–25.
4. Otterman S. 'I trust science,' Says nurse who is first to get vaccine in U.S. In: New York times. Available at: https://www.nytimes.com/2020/12/14/nyregion/us-covid-vaccine-first-sandra-lindsay.html. Accessed August 17, 2022.
5. Fahrenwald NL, Bassett SD, Tschetter L, et al. Teaching core nursing values. J Prof Nurs 2005;21(1):46–51.
6. Shaw HK, Degazon C. Integrating the core professional values of nursing: a profession, not just a career. J Cult Divers 2008;15(1):44–50.
7. Aubrey A. Sandra Lindsay got the first U.S. COVID jab. Here's her secret to motivate others. NPR: Shots. Available at: https://www.npr.org/sections/health-shots/

2021/12/13/1063020183/sandra-lindsay-got-the-first-u-s-covid-jab-heres-her-secret-to-motivate-others. Accessed August 19, 2022.

8. The Woodhull Study on nursing and the media: health care's invisible partner. Revolution 1998;8(2):64–70.

9. Mason DJ, Nixon L, Glickstein B, et al. The woodhull study revisited: nurses' representation in health news media 20 years later. J Nurs Scholarsh 2018;50(6): 695–704. https://doi.org/10.1111/jnu.12429.

10. Saad L. Military brass, judges among professions at new image lows. In: Gallup. Available at: https://news.gallup.com/poll/388649/military-brass-judges-among-professions-new- image-lows.aspx. Accessed August 17, 2022.

11. Confronting Health Misinformation. The U.S. surgeon general's advisory on building a healthy information environment. Available at: https://www.hhs.gov/sites/default/files/surgeon-general-misinformation-advisory.pdf. Accessed August 22, 2022.

12. Garcia R, Qureshi I. Nurse identity: reality and media portrayal. Evid Based Nurs 2022;25(1):1–5.

13. Teresa-Morales C, Rodríguez-Pérez M, Araujo-Hernández M, et al. Current stereotypes associated with nursing and nursing professionals: an integrative review. Int J Environ Res 2022;19(13):7640.

14. Social media. Merriam-Webster. Available at: https://www.merriam-webster.com/dictionary/social%20media. Accessed August 25, 2022.

15. Myers CR. Promoting population health: nurse advocacy, policy making, and use of media. Nurs Clin North Am 2020;55(1):11–20.

16. Nurses Make Change Happen. National Nurse-Led Care Consortium a PHMC Affiliate. Available at: https://vaccinetoolkit.phmc.org/. Accessed August 22, 2022.

17. Centers for Disease Control and Prevention. COVID data tracker. Atlanta, GA: US Department of Health and Human Services, CDC; 2022. Available at: https://covid.cdc.gov/covid-data-tracker.

18. KFF COVID-19 Vaccine Monitor, KFF. Available at: https://www.kff.org/coronavirus-covid-19/dashboard/kff-covid-19-vaccine-monitor-dashboard/. Accessed August 19, 2022.

19. Dong E, Du H, Gardner L. An interactive web-based dashboard to track COVID-19 in real time. Lancet Infect Dis 2020;20(5):P533–4.

20. Bonnevie E, Rosenberg SD, Kummeth C, et al. Using social media influencers to increase knowledge and positive attitudes toward the flu vaccine. PLoS One 2020;15(10):e0240828.

21. Irvine M. Google Ads Benchmarks for YOUR Industry [Updated!]. WordStream by LOCALiQ. Available at: https://www.wordstream.com/blog/ws/2016/02/29/google-adwords-industry-benchmarks. Accessed August 18, 2022.

22. Chan AKM, Nickson CP, Rudolph JW, et al. Social media for rapid knowledge dissemination: early experience from the COVID-19 pandemic. Anaesthesia 2020;75(12):1579–82.

23. Epstein B, Turner M. The nursing code of ethics: its value, its history. Online J Issues Nurs 2015;20(2):4.

24. McCartney P. Social networking principles for nurses. MCN. Am J Maternal/Child Nurs 2012;37(2):131.

Out of Chaos Leaders Emerged

Petra Brysiewicz, PhD[a],*, Jennifer Chipps, PhD[b]

KEYWORDS

- Leadership • Nursing • Resilience • COVID-19

KEY POINTS

- COVID-19 had a major influence on nursing highlighting the indispensable role played by nurses.
- The chaos of the pandemic resulted in real physical and emotional risks to nurses.
- Challenges of moral distress, fear for self and family, and work impact were common.
- In the face of all these challenges, nurses demonstrated extraordinary resilience, leadership, and innovation.
- Nursing emerged from the pandemic with visible leadership in the field of health.

INTRODUCTION

There has always been a recognition for the need of a strong nursing workforce in history. After the end of World War II, President Truman in the Associated Press, 1946, February 28, stated that nurses are "one of the most important groups of health workers in the country."[1] More than 70 years later, in 2020, the Year of the Nurse, with more than 5 million cases of COVID-19 recorded around the world, "nurses were standing firm against the onslaught of the virus and have saved many thousands of lives" (ICN President, 2020).[2]

Toward the end of 2019, our world changed due to the COVID-19 pandemic, and our lives, both personally and professionally, were irrevocably altered. Although hailed as heroes,[3] nurses were faced with finding new ways of living and new ways of working while navigating this changed landscape. For nurses across the globe, numerous new challenges emerged but so too has there been the emergence of a resilient workforce with new learning and ways of doing.

[a] School of Nursing & Public Health, University of KwaZulu-Natal, King George Mazisi Kunene Road, Glenwood, Durban 4041, South Africa; [b] School of Nursing, Faculty of Community and Health Sciences, University of the Western Cape, 14 Blanckenberg Road, Belville, Cape Town 7041, South Africa
* Corresponding author.
E-mail address: brysiewiczp@ukzn.ac.za
Twitter: @PetraBrysiewicz (P.B.)

Nurs Clin N Am 58 (2023) 87–96
https://doi.org/10.1016/j.cnur.2022.10.006
0029-6465/23/© 2022 Elsevier Inc. All rights reserved.

COVID-19 has done a great deal to globally highlight the indispensable role played by nurses within the health-care system and has served to assist to address the invisibility of nurses, despite their limited voice in the national and regional responses to the COVID-19 pandemic.[4] Nurses have always been the backbone of the workforce, doing phenomenal and unbelievable work daily as they save lives, prevent complications, and prevent suffering, often unnoticed.[1] Nurses' stories from all corners of the world need to be written and exposed to the world because nurses have a plethora of wisdom to get out there. Through the chaos, COVID-19 has provided an opportunity to "tell these stories."

"Unpacking" THE CHAOS OF THE PANDEMIC

During the last 50 years, health-care workers, and specifically nurses, have encountered numerous risks from HIV/AIDS, SARS, swine flu, and Ebola.[5] Although COVID-19 was thought not to be as deadly as HIV/AIDS or the swine flu, the insufficient understanding of the virus at the start of the pandemic, its pathophysiology, mode of transmission, susceptibility profile, and contagious nature along with failures in the supply chains for personal protective equipment (PPE) meant that health-care workers were asked to take on substantial but uncertain risk.[5]

Challenges Related to Physical and Emotional Risks of COVID-19

These uncertain risks have had a large impact on the nursing workforce. It has been reported that the health workforce had a 7 times higher risk of severe COVID-19 infection compared with other workers.[6] The World Health Organization estimated that a possible 115,500 health-care workers have died from COVID-19 in the period between January 2020 to May 2021,[7] although the real impact has remained unknown.[8] The uncertainty and the real risk faced by nurses on a daily basis resulted in high levels of COVID-19 fear related to infection and safety concerns for themselves and their families,[9] as well as work burnout with emotional exhaustion, depression,[9] and possible posttraumatic stress. In a study conducted in South Africa, nearly half of the nurses included in the study were extremely concerned about family members and their own personal health[10] with 3 in 5 nurses concerned about passing the infection on to family members.[10] Qualitative stories globally from nurses also identified themes such as the shock of the virus, staff sacrifice and dedication, as well as collateral damage ranging from personal health concerns to the long-term impact on, and the care of, discharged patients and a hierarchy of power and inequality within the health-care system.[11]

Moral Distress and Ethical Challenges

One of the hidden challenges faced by nurses during the pandemic was the moral distress experienced in scenarios such as witnessing and participating in the triaging of resources and equipment to those who were seen as having a better chance of survival; watching patients dying alone without their family or loved ones due to visitor restrictions and social isolation policies; experiencing the cumulative loss of high number of patient deaths; suffering from physical exhaustion due to a heavy workload, schedule changes and shifting roles; experiencing anxieties about limited medical supplies, equipment, hospital beds, and PPE; and struggling with worry about their own health and possible exposure of their families while balancing professional obligation.[12,13] Although for nurses from low-to-middle-income countries, having to make very difficult patient-management decisions according to the availability of resources is often a daily occurrence, for many in other higher income countries, this was a new reality never previously experienced. Nurses also faced several ethical challenges[14] due to the conflicting professional values and unpalatable and complex ethical issues in practice.[15] Nurses were placed in situations where the professional values of protecting the public from harm and a duty to provide care were in conflict with obligations to protect own health and the health of families[15] all the while addressing equity of care issues in terms of triaging care, and patients not expected to survive but still needing care with the fair allocation of resources.[12] Faced with the potential reality that patients will suffer, clinically deteriorate, or die, many health-care professionals found it extremely difficult to make or implement a decision to deny or delay treatment given their own human response, their professional socialization, and their profession's expectations and norms about saving lives, relieving suffering, and not abandoning patients.[15]

Challenges of COVID Stigma

Another challenge experienced in many countries by nurses and other health-care professionals was that of COVID-19 stigma. In Malawi, nurses were not allowed to use public transport and were insulted in the street and evicted from rented apartments,[16] and a nurse from Mexico was sprayed with bleach.[17] A study in Italy found that nurses experienced "stigma in the working environment" such as avoiding closeness with others, and "stigma in everyday life" with strong feelings of isolation because people avoided contact.[18] In May 2020, a community of advocates from 13 medical and humanitarian organizations issued a declaration condemning more than 200 incidents of COVID-19–related attacks on health-care professionals and health facilities during the ongoing pandemic.[16] This was happening at the same time as public displays of affection such as "clapping for hospital workers"[3] (**Box 1**). This concern regarding the stigma for nurses associated with working in COVID-19 was highlighted by the International Council of Nurses, which called on governments internationally to stop attacks on nurses.[19]

Facing Challenges with Resilience

However, amid this chaos and challenges, nurses have demonstrated extraordinary resilience. COVID-19 forced nurses to come up with new ways to manage and respond to the pandemic: to be quick to act appropriately, to be alert to changes that are needed, and to be receptive and adaptable to change. During the pandemic, many retired nurses returned to the workforce to assist as needed, undertaking further training to work in contact-tracing, COVID-testing stations, testing work, and in specialized units such as intensive care units (ICUs) and emergency departments.[20]

Nurses working with COVID-19 patients were reported to have significantly greater resilience than other nurses[21] and front-line nurses experienced both positive and negative impacts of COVID-19, with the positive impact reported as increased empathy, compassion, and enhanced confidence in their professional skills.[22] In a study in China, 96.8% of the nurses expressed their frontline work willingness, and 60.6% reported a sense of personal accomplishment working during COVID-19.[9] Research has indicated that nurses tended to adopt positive strategies in the face of the psychological impact of the pandemic.[23] This is in support with what Bonano[24] in 2004 suggested, namely that understanding what you are doing, having a meaningful purpose and a strong belief system helped people become more resilient in stressful situations.[25] "*Showing stubborn hope*,"[26] moral courage, stamina and resilience, nurses continued to work on the front lines of the pandemic, once again holding the historic center of the recognition, prevention, care and control of infectious diseases from the time of Florence Nightingale.[15]

Box 1
Some of the challenges experienced by nurses during COVID-19

Fear for self and family
• Dealing with a new unknown pandemic
• Constant fear due to caring for patients not yet tested
• Fear of infection from patients and work colleagues
• Increased susceptibility to major health issues due to preexisting health issues
• Fear of transmission to family and loved ones
• Physical exhaustion
• Resulting psychological stress, burnout, and traumatic stress disorder (PTSD)

Work challenges
• Excessive job stress and constant high work pressure
• Constantly changing workplace policies and procedures
• Role and task shifting, for example, having to work in role not trained for
• Large crowds of patients entering the workplace with COVID-19 and needing further space and resources
• Trying to do more without additional resources, often in an already high-pressure low-resourced environment (especially problematic in Low- and Middle-income Countries [LMIC])
• Working a busy shift in full PPE (if available)—impact on skin and added difficulties in communication and establishing rapport with patients
• Having to deal with a lot of emotions from patients and their families
• Not allowing visitors and or families to be present, often resulting in conflict

Ethical and Moral challenges
• Modification of admission criteria and triaging resources
• Withdrawing treatment due to resource constraints
• Facilitating final goodbye's with families excluded from the bedside
• Shortages of isolation rooms and equipment
• Feeling underprepared to function within the allocated role

Community challenges
• Managing expectations of community members
• Stigma toward health-care workers
• COVID-19 conspiracy theories

OUT OF THE CHAOS, NURSES AS LEADERS EMERGE

However, in this chaos, we found the emergence of stories of innovation and successes in nursing care. Drawing inspiration from a Xhosa word used in South Africa—*zenzele*—which refers to the need to do things on your own without relying on others to do it for you, the COVID-19 pandemic has seen nurses across the globe taking up the initiative. They have recognized the need, realized there is nothing in place to assist and have thus risen to the challenge to provide a solution. These solutions have been in the form of innovative practices, communication and support strategies to assist the communities they serve.

Nurse Innovations in Clinical Practice

The pandemic caused a great many challenges in the clinical area thereby providing the impetus and forcing organizations, and specifically nurses, to think creatively and to be a valuable contributor to the multidisciplinary health-care team.[27] Nurses have a rich tradition of being recognized as the "hackers of the hospital," that is, working creatively to solve issues of patient care, customizing medical equipment, and making new devices to ensure patient comfort and safety.[28,29] There are numerous examples of this from across the world and include something as simple as a

Table 1	
Some examples of COVID-19 nurse innovations from around the world	
Innovation	**Description of Its Application in the Clinical Area**
Own photograph on the front of your gown	Masks and face shields hide the face and facial expressions of the nurse. Photographs of the nurse's face with their first name was attached and displayed to the front of their gown for patients to be able to see who was taking care of them
"Real Talk Real Time"	This virtual rounding tool has been able to provide comfort to family members by allowing them to be face-to-face with their loved one's nurses or doctors in the ICU. Unlike other video chat offerings, using the Webex platform ensured it was secure and able to be accessed on multiple devices by various age groups. https://nursing.jnj.com/nursing-news-events/nurses-leading-innovation/meet-10-nurses-pioneering-innovative-covid-19-solutions
"Code Cards" with most commonly coded medications and procedures	These communication cards are used in isolation rooms, where they are held up to the glass to get important messages to the rest of the team (about required medication) during a resuscitation, thereby keeping the staff safe. https://nursing.jnj.com/nursing-news-events/nurses-leading-innovation/meet-10-nurses-pioneering-innovative-covid-19-solutions
IsoPouch (Isolation Pouch)	This was created by a nurse who realized the need for an inexpensive disposable pouch that she could fill with all the supplies she needed to care for her isolated patients, and which she could then throw away with her gown and other PPE once finished[30]
Handover Redesign Team	Nurse leaders and clinical nurses redesigned the bedside handover, and this was carried out in order to improve nursing practice implementation and handover processes that addressed nursing concerns and prioritized their needs[31]
"Hand of God"—water-filled nonsterile glove	This is placed in the hand of an intubated and ventilated patient, allowing them the feeling that someone is nearby, with them, holding their hand. This was in response to COVID-19 social distancing rules that families were not allowed at the bedside

photograph attached to a nurses gown (**Table 1**), an inflated nonsterile glove nestled in the hand of a sedated and ventilated patient, to the "Real talk Real time" virtual tool (see **Table 1**). COVID-19 also changed the way in which nurses at the bedside could practice. Nurses worked to find simple and cost effective practical solutions to many of these challenges, see "Isopouch" and "Code Cards" (see **Table 1**), while still providing support and high-quality care within the tight constraints of isolation and working effectively, despite increasing numbers of patients, by improving bedside handover as patient numbers surged (see **Table 1**).

Digital innovation has always been present in the clinical areas and well used by the bedside nurse, however, possibly not to its full potential. COVID-19 challenged that[32] and resulted in numerous innovations in the clinical setting. The global pandemic accelerated the pace of this technological innovation across the entire world with, for example, mobile apps being used for monitoring quarantine in Sierra Leone and South Africa, information-providing drones in place in Rwanda,[33] and using social media such as WhatsApp for support, information, and communication.

Innovation is about using one's own knowledge and skills to change old ways of thinking and practicing and to develop new improved ways of working.[34] This can be an extremely challenging task, and it is essential to be very purposive about the way in which we are educating nurses and to ensure we are adequately preparing them for success in the fourth industrial revolution. An additional problem is, however, that nurse innovations such as these often remain "hidden" because they do not spread beyond the area in which they were developed. This is for a variety of reasons including the limited dissemination of such products in written articles. This is especially true for lower income countries such as those in Africa, where many young scientists face numerous challenges converting their research into publications.[35] Gomez-Marquez and Young (2016) argue that, "It is time to not only acknowledge nurses' creativity and ingenuity, but celebrate and nurture it."[28] In order for innovation to thrive however, it needs a supportive environment. It is also important to reflect on the question, "What are we doing to nurture and support nurse innovation?"

Communication Innovations

Communication became a central concern during the COVID-19 pandemic due to social distancing policies, the use of full PPE, and the novelty of the disease. This was particularly true regarding the ways in which nurses interacted with patients' families, with significant restrictions on visiting and face-to-face consultations.[36] Nurses found new ways to communicate effectively with patients, family, and colleagues, by adapting to virtual consultations.[20] WhatsApp collaboration groups with staff members and in ICUs by linking families with video iPad sessions to see their loved ones. This was evident in ICUs in the National Health Service (United Kingdom), where interactions with families were handled with video calling used in 63 (47%) of the ICUs and 39 (29%) ICUs had developed a dedicated family communication team.[36] In South Africa, provincial departments of health established collaborative learning environments—#Colabs—as a learning space. This served to provide a space in which to share experiences, insights, and ideas that then translated to improvements in different clinical settings, including supporting staff. These #Colabs also played a valuable role in providing professional recognition for innovations in practices.[37] These included "*daily walkabouts*" by nurse leadership to ask frontline staff every day "what matters to you" and then to act daily with "*just do it*" quick fixes to address identified challenges. "*Daily huddles*" were virtual daily get-togethers, which served to establish 2-way communication through WhatsApp to broadcast rapidly changing polices, actions, and successes of frontline worker stories.[37]

Innovations for support and fostering resilience

During the pandemic, nurse leaders contributed to many original solutions that limited the spread of disease and aided the pandemic response while supporting rapid changes across health systems in keeping with changing local and national policies, emerging data trends, scientific discoveries, and surge capacity requirements.[38] The resilience of staff to swiftly adapt to this new, uncertain landscape of nursing and patient care was essential and leadership needed to continue to work toward engaging nurses at the bedside to ensure best practices and resilient nurses.[31] Leadership through a crisis is essential for the protective effect of nurses' emotional well-being and learning from the pandemic about the impact of leadership in a crisis is important to facilitate recovery and lessen the impact in further outbreaks.[39] Nurse leadership stepped up to create working environments that not only supports individual resilience but also organizational resilience. Nursing practice is conducted within an environment influenced and shaped by leaders, and recognizing the limits of individual resilience and a nurse's capacity to manage chronic levels of physical, emotional, and moral distress is essential. Nursing leadership promoted strategies to enhance organizational resilience during and beyond the pandemic by creating an environment of trust and psychological safety, supporting nurse empowerment, and nurturing communication structures.[40] To foster and preserve organizational resilience, leaders have to identify the challenges, ensure that workplace structures and processes are in place, and if they are not, they needed to advocate for them[40] and consider employing different leadership styles to support nurse's well-being.[39]

THE EMERGENCE OF VISIBLE NURSE LEADERSHIP

The COVID-19 pandemic thus brought with it many examples of complete disorder and confusion for individuals, communities, societies, and the world at large, and although nursing has risen to the challenge, suffered a great deal along the way, the pandemic has also provided great opportunities for the profession. COVID-19 has exposed the truth about nursing more than any organized campaign could have possibly done. It brought to light nursing's indispensable role as the backbone of the health-care system and has highlighted their professionalism, not only as frontline care providers but also as health-care leaders and policy experts. It has provided an unprecedented opportunity for the general public to witness firsthand the vital role that nurses play.[20] The question for nursing now is whether to continue in our roles as implementers of policies that are handed to us or to use our size and influence for representation in places where decision-making that affects our practice, welfare, and profession are being discussed.[20]

Nursing leadership needs to be visible and must play an active role in multidisciplinary and interprofessional collaborative decision-making. Nurses have unique health-care expertise, and it is vital that they have a voice not only in high-level decision-making about the response and planning for the COVID-19 pandemic but also in future health crises.[4] Nurse leaders need to be adaptive and strategic while demonstrating concern regarding the well-being of the nursing workforce.[41]

SUMMARY

COVID-19 is nothing like we ever could have anticipated, and it has irrevocably changed the world as we know it. This includes the nursing profession and has resulted in fundamental changes to the way in which nurses work. Nurses have been thrust into this challenging situation and have been called on to play a large and extremely important role in the management of this pandemic while still struggling for meaningful recognition as professionals on the frontline of the pandemic. It is also important that the leadership, the innovations, and resilience stories are shared and made visible through publication and professional recognition of the pivotal role of nurses in health. This is an opportunity to highlight to the world the value of nursing, the contribution of nursing, to increase the visibility of nursing and the phenomenal work that nurses do. So *"let's not waste a good disaster."*

CLINICS CARE POINTS

- Provide clear and visible responsive leadership at all times
- Clear transparent communication during a crisis with all stakeholders, including health workers and families, is paramount
- Create working environments of trust and safety

DISCLOSURE

The authors have nothing to disclose.

REFERENCES

1. Edmonds JK, Kneipp SM, Campbell L. A call to action for public health nurses during the COVID-19 pandemic. Public Health Nurs 2020;37(3):323.
2. ICN highlights top priorities to beat COVID-19. Available at: https://www.icn.ch/news/icn-highlights-top-priorities-beat-covid-19.
3. Chipps J, Jarvis MA, Brysiewicz P. Heroes and angels: ED nurses' ongoing fight for meaningful recognition as professionals on the frontline of the pandemic. Int Emerg Nurs 2021;59:101080.
4. Rasmussen B, Holton S, Wynter K, et al. We're on mute! Exclusion of nurses' voices in national decisions and responses to COVID-19: An international perspective. J Adv Nurs 2022;78(7):e87–90.
5. Morley G, Grady C, McCarthy J, et al. Covid-19: Ethical challenges for nurses. Hastings Cent Rep 2020;50(3):35–9.
6. Mutambudzi M, Niedzwiedz C, Macdonald EB, et al. Occupation and risk of severe COVID-19: prospective cohort study of 120 075 UK Biobank participants. Occup Environ Med 2021;78(5):307.
7. World Health Organization. The impact of COVID-19 on health and care workers: a closer look at deaths.. 2021. https://apps.who.int/iris/handle/10665/345300.
8. The toll of COVID-19 on health care workers remains unknown. Am J Nurs 2021; 121(3):14–5.
9. Hu D, Kong Y, Li W, et al. Frontline nurses' burnout, anxiety, depression, and fear statuses and their associated factors during the COVID-19 outbreak in Wuhan, China: a large-scale cross-sectional study. EClinicalMedicine 2020;24:100424.
10. HSRC. *Survey of COVD-19*, South African Healthworkers. 2020. Available at: htpp:/www.hsrc.ac.a/news/media-and-covid19.
11. Bennett P, Noble S, Johnston S, et al. COVID-19 confessions: a qualitative exploration of healthcare workers experiences of working with COVID-19. BMJ Open 2020;10(12):e043949.
12. Greenberg N, Docherty M, Gnanapragasam S, et al. Managing mental health challenges faced by healthcare workers during covid-19 pandemic. BMJ 2020; 368:m1211.
13. Talevi D, Socci V, Carai M, et al. Mental health outcomes of the CoViD-19 pandemic. Rivista di psichiatria 2020;55(3):137–44.

14. Robert R, Kentish-Barnes N, Boyer A, et al. Ethical dilemmas due to the Covid-19 pandemic. Ann Intensive Care 2020;10(1):1–9.

15. Turale S, Meechamnan C, Kunaviktikul W. Challenging times: ethics, nursing and the COVID-19 pandemic. Int Nurs Rev 2020;67(2):164–7.

16. Bagcchi S. Stigma during the COVID-19 pandemic. Lancet Infect Dis 2020; 20(7):782.

17. Health workers become unexpected targets during covid-19. Economist 2021. Available at: https://www.economist.com/international/2020/05/11/health-workers-become-unexpected-targets-during-covid-19.

18. Simeone S, Rea T, Guillari A, et al. Nurses and stigma at the time of covid-19: A phenomenological study. MDPI 2021;10(1):25.

19. ICN calls for government action to stop attacks on nurses at a time when their mental health and wellbeing are already under threat because of COVID-19 pandemic. 2020. Available at: https://www.icn.ch/news/icn-calls-government-action-stop-attacks-nurses-time-when-their-mental-health-and-wellbeing.

20. Popoola T. COVID-19's missing heroes: Nurses' contribution and visibility in Aotearoa New Zealand. Nurs Praxis Aotearoa New Zealand 2021;37.

21. Jo S, Kurt S, Bennett JA, et al. Nurses' resilience in the face of coronavirus (COVID-19): An international view. Nurs Health Sci 2021;23(3):646–57.

22. Tan R, Yu T, Luo K, et al. Experiences of clinical first-line nurses treating patients with COVID-19: A qualitative study. Journal of Nurs Manage 2020;28(6):1381–90.

23. Sierra-García E, Sosa-Palanca EM, Saus-Ortega C, et al. Modulating elements of nurse resilience in population care during the COVID-19 pandemic. Int J Environ Res Public Health 2022;19(8):4452.

24. Bonanno GA. Loss, trauma, and human resilience: have we underestimated the human capacity to thrive after extremely aversive events? Am Psychol 2004; 59(1):20.

25. Duncan DL. What the COVID-19 pandemic tells us about the need to develop resilience in the nursing workforce. Nurs Manage 2020;27(3).

26. Coetzee S, Klopper H, Jansen J. In our own words: nurses on the front line. South Africa: Jonathan Ball Publishers; 2022.

27. Wymer JA, Stucky CH, De Jong MJ. Nursing leadership and COVID-19: defining the shadows and leading ahead of the data. Nurse Lead 2021;19(5):483–8.

28. Gomez-Marquez J, Young A. A history of nurse making and stealth innovation. Available at SSRN 2778663. 2016.

29. Thomas TW, Seifert PC, Joyner JC. Registered nurses leading innovative changes. OJIN 2016;21(3):3.

30. Rabbitt M. COVID-19 inspired me to improve patient care": how two nurses devised new ways to help kids and fellow nurses during the pandemic. 2021. https://www.jnj.com/innovation/how-covid-19-inspired-nurses-to-innovate-improve-patient-care?_amp=true.

31. Brown-Deveaux D, Kaplan S, Gabbe L, et al. Transformational leadership meets innovative strategy: how nurse leaders and clinical nurses redesigned bedside handover to improve nursing practice. Nurse Leader 2022;20(3):290–6.

32. Horton T, Hardie T, Mahadeva S, et al. Securing a positive health care technology legacy from COVID-19. London: Health Foundation; 2021.

33. Andersen, H. 2020. Insights From Africa's Covid-19 Response: Tech Innovations. Available at: https://institute.global/advisory/insights-africas-covid-19-response-tech-innovations Accessed December 10, 2020.

34. Brysiewicz P, Hughes TL, McCreary LL. Promoting innovation in global nursing practice. Rwanda J 2015;2(2):41–5.

35. Kumwenda S, El Hadji AN, Orondo PW, et al. Challenges facing young African scientists in their research careers: A qualitative exploratory study. Malawi Med J 2017;29(1):1–4.
36. Boulton AJ, Jordan H, Adams CE, et al. Intensive care unit visiting and family communication during the COVID-19 pandemic: A UK survey. J Intensive Care Soc 2021;23(3):293–6, 17511437211007779.
37. Staff CARE #Colab. Available at: https://community.ihi.org/za/provinces/westerncape.
38. Daly J, Jackson D, Anders R, et al. Who speaks for nursing? COVID-19 highlighting gaps in leadership. J Clin Nurs 2020;29(15–16):2751–2.
39. Phillips N, Hughes L, Vindrola-Padros C, et al. The impact of leadership on the nursing workforce during the COVID-10 pandemic. BMJ Leader; 2022.
40. Udod S, MacPhee M, Baxter P. Rethinking resilience: nurses and nurse leaders emerging from the post–covid-19 environment. JONA 2021;51(11):537–40.
41. Rosser E, Buckner E, Avedissian T, et al. The global leadership mentoring community: building capacity across seven global regions. Int Nurs Rev 2020;67(4):484–94.

Using Technology to Facilitate Evidence-Based Practice During the COVID-19 Pandemic

Philip D. Walker, MLIS, MS[a], Catherine H. Ivory, PhD, RN-BC, NEA-BC[b],*

KEYWORDS

- Information needs • Information seeking behavior • Nursing • Infodemic
- Information overload • COVID-19

KEY POINTS

- Identify a single point of access to reduce information seeking barriers (time, searching skills, resource awareness).
- Creating saved search strings tailored to nursing interests enables efficient access to relevant information.
- Monitor the literature and revise search strings accordingly.
- Use a team-based approach to reduce workload, burden, and increase scalability.

INTRODUCTION

Infectious disease outbreaks or epidemics can appear very suddenly and with little to no notice. Whether the etiological organism is novel or familiar, these abrupt public health events can immediately overwhelm the local or national health care infrastructure and the health care workforce. Nurses' roles as frontline staff are particularly prone to anxiety and burnout due to clinical uncertainty and the feeling of being unprepared, powerless, and frightened for their health and families.[1-6] Studies from previous global infectious disease outbreaks, epidemics, or pandemics (human immunodeficiency virus [HIV]/AIDS, influenza, Ebola, severe acute respiratory syndrome [SARS], Middle East respiratory syndrome [MERS]) and the current COVID-19 pandemic illustrate the importance of timely delivery of information pertaining to protocols, guidelines, precautionary measures, identifying and avoiding risks, and

[a] Annette and Irwin Eskind Family Biomedical Library and Learning Center, Vanderbilt University, 2209 Garland Avenue, Nashville, TN 37240, USA; [b] Practice Excellence, Vanderbilt University Medical Center, 2611 West End Avenue, Suite 328, Nashville, TN 37203, USA
* Corresponding author.
E-mail address: cathy.ivory@vumc.org
Twitter: @civoryrnc (C.H.I.)

Nurs Clin N Am 58 (2023) 97–106
https://doi.org/10.1016/j.cnur.2022.10.009
0029-6465/23/© 2022 Elsevier Inc. All rights reserved.

overall safety.[1,4,7–10] This information is traditionally derived from trusted sources such as federal agencies, Ministries of Health, and the World Health Organization.[9,11] The timing, content, and mechanisms of disseminating outbreak-related information are empowering; instill a sense of control and confidence; improve the ability to cope; and reduce psychological distress, anxiety, fear, confusion, error, and spreading of misinformation.[7,12]

Since January 2020, the world has been saturated with information related to the novel coronavirus, severe acute respiratory syndrome-COV-2, SARS-COV-2, or the more popular term, COVID-19. Information is disseminated from local, state, national, and international health authorities, governments, print and visual media news outlets, businesses, organizations, educational institutions, and countless social media platforms. Nurses were experiencing information overload long before the COVID-19 pandemic[13,14] but current information and communication technologies increased the amount of available information exponentially and with less effort.[15] Evidence derived from biomedical research and clinical practice is essential for improving health care safety, quality, and efficiency. When the pandemic began, evidence was badly needed. However, the information or evidence ecosystem was perceived as being in constant disarray during the pandemic.[15–22]

The issues surrounding nursing and evidence-based practice have been investigated, discussed, and are well documented.[23] As previously stated, the COVID-19 pandemic exacerbated those issues due to the amount of information generated and the constant changing of preventative measures and treatment guidance disseminated to health care providers. However, it is interesting to note that only a small percentage of preventative and treatment guidance can be considered research evidence and an even smaller amount applied to the varied information needs of nurses. A broad Medline (via PubMed) search (performed June 30, 2022) on COVID-19 yields 272,667 results. However, as shown in **Table 1**, less than 0.07% of the COVID-19 literature in the Medline database was research evidence. The nursing-specific literature base was even more sparse and remains so today. When the pandemic began, nurses needed the best available evidence quickly and in a format that was consumable.

To combat the known barriers to evidence-based practice, the investigators discussed the need for a technological solution to provide nurses with efficient access to the biomedical literature, particularly to topics that may not be addressed in standard governmental, organizational, or association communications. This article discusses the development of a Web-based platform composed of saved search strings in the Medline database (PubMed) and other vetted information resources pertaining to the COVID-19 pandemic.

BACKGROUND

Similar to many hospitals and health systems, our academic medical center created a COVID-19 Command Center in March, 2020. Initially, the command center focused on planning for the nursing care needs for the influx of patients seeking COVID-19 testing or treatment. Operational and research colleagues modeled various scenarios based on trends of COVID-19 spread in other countries and its arrival in the United States; nursing operations projected staffing needs based on this modeling. Nursing stakeholders and the local health department planned alternate locations for patients should existing acute care beds be full. We organized COVID-19 testing locations to minimize exposure and risk. We created contingency plans for staffing that included mobilizing additional clinical nurses who were currently working in nonclinical roles. We monitored supplies of personal protective equipment (PPE) and updated PPE

Table 1 Medline (PubMed) evidence-based practice search results		
	Limits (January 1, 2020– June 30, 2022)	Number of Results (%)
COVID-19	None	272,667
COVID-19	Evidence publication types[a]	18,336 (0.07)
COVID-19 AND nurse[a]	None	16,606 (0.06)
COVID-19 AND nurse[a]	Evidence publication types[a]	1275 (0.005)

[a] NOTE: PubMed EBM search filters: clinical trial, comparative study, controlled clinical trial, guidelines, meta-analysis, multicenter study, observational study, practice guidelines, randomized clinical trial, systematic review.

use policies. Visitor policies were modified. Student clinical rotations moved from onsite to simulated experiences. Telehealth services expanded. Workers, including nurses who were not at the bedside, began working remotely. Because COVID-19 was a novel virus, little was definitively known about how best to protect against it or how best to treat it. The medical center's office of evidence-based practice (EBP) and nursing research wanted to provide the best available evidence to nursing teams to use for decision making.

APPROACH

We (CI, PW) met virtually on April 3, 2020 to discuss opportunities to collate evidence-based practice resources into an interface useful for bedside nurses, nursing leaders, and nursing faculty. A prototype was developed by using the LibGuides (SpringShare, Miami, FL, USA) platform, including several of the recent searches performed by one of us (PW). After reviewing the prototype, authors agreed upon a few minor edits and finalized an initial set of search topics and Web resources that were perceived to be relevant and specific to nursing. Because of the urgency of COVID-19 information needs, the project's user template and search topics were communicated to the biomedical library's Information Services Team to expedite its development. The resulting *Nursing EBP for COVID-19* Webpage, https://researchguides.library.vanderbilt.edu/COVID19ebp, was given top-level placement on the Eskind Biomedical Library's homepage (**Fig. 1**). The biomedical library's Web portal was already a well-known, respected, and highly used resource; thus, this new, central point of access did not require any additional permissions or health information technology resources. Once live, the Web portal was promoted through the previously mentioned Command Center. After the initial national lockdown period, our shared governance committees began meeting virtually, which provided additional opportunities to promote these evidence-based resources through shared governance committees, especially clinical practice committees. There were also links to the biomedical library interface included on other nursing Web sites across the enterprise.

Additional topics were added from search requests by the adult academic health center's clinical practice committee, as well as any pressing issues deemed valuable by the library team. The primary objective was to create and save search strings (**Fig. 2**) on topics specifically related to COVID-19 but its novelty resulted in a shortage of relevant literature. An opportune discovery in PubMed uncovered numerous research articles on the experience of nurses caring for patients during other infectious diseases and other pandemics, including HIV/AIDS, Ebola, Zika virus, SARS, MERS,

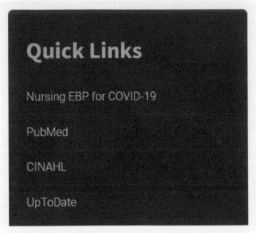

Fig. 1. Eskind library home page quick links.

and H1N1 influenza. Many of these articles were international studies but yielded insightful information in the absence of COVID-19 literature. Thus, all searches were duplicated but supplemented with broader search terms such as "epidemics," "pandemics," "infectious disease outbreaks," and the aforementioned diseases. As the COVID-19 research literature began to increase in availability, it was vital to begin providing tips and training on how to revise, refine, and tailor searches to bring

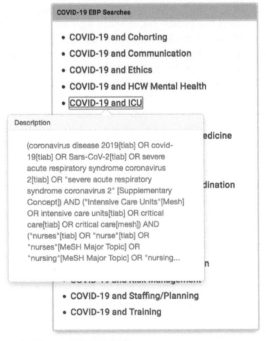

Fig. 2. Covid-19 EBP pubMed search example.

efficiencies to information seeking and knowledge translation. The Webpage for the office of EBP and Nursing Research included tips about how to refine search results and members of the Information Services Team provided individual instruction upon request on how to refine and revise the existing search strings.

FINAL CONTENT AND USAGE ANALYSIS

The final *Nursing EBP for COVID-19* Webpage consists of 38 saved searches (17 COVID-19, 19 Epidemics/Pandemics, 2 EBP search strings; limited to clinical trials, guidelines, systematic reviews, meta-analyses) and 18 curated links to vetted resources from professional associations, library vendors, US governmental agencies, and international bodies. The full list of search topics is listed in **Fig. 3**. The Webpage had a total of 3129 views from April 2020 to June 2022, averaging 116 views each month. The highest use period was April 2020 to March 2021, with more than 100 Webpage views each month. The range of monthly views during that high use period was 105 to 356. Usage has remained constant but reduced since October 2021.

The most searched topics (from highest to lowest) are Nursing, Infection Control, Nursing Research, Patient Care, and Personal Protective Equipment (**Table 2**). These topics coincide with what has been presented in previous epidemic/pandemic related literature. From an informatics and administrative perspective, if research suggests these topics are highly valued by nurses, then further investigation is warranted, in order to be more proactive with dissemination of this type of clinical information and the generation of new knowledge, in order to be prepared for the next infectious disease outbreak.

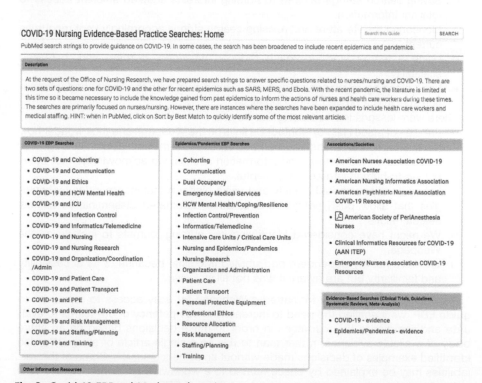

Fig. 3. Covid-19 EBP pubMed search topics.

Table 2	
Most popular PubMed search topics	
Most Used Links (March 2020–June 2022)	
Topic	Total
COVID-19 and Nursing	347
COVID-19 and Infection Control	299
COVID-19 and Nursing Research	215
COVID-19 and Patient Care	188
COVID-19 and PPE	138
COVID-19 and ICU	114
COVID-19 and Patient Cohorting	100
COVID-19 and Health Care Worker Mental Health	88
COVID-19 Evidence-Based Search Filters	77
COVID-19 and Communication	74
COVID-19 and Staffing/Planning	74

DISCUSSION

Here is a summary of what worked well with the technology solution:

a. Creating a single point of access to reduce information seeking barriers (time, searching skills, resource awareness).

b. Saving search strings tailored to nursing interests enabled efficient access to relevant information.

c. Monitoring the literature and revising search strings accordingly kept resources current.

d. Using a team-based approach reduced workload, burden, and increased scalability.

e. Long-standing relationships and established trust with the library and information specialists proved to be beneficial.

There were lessons learned along the way:

f. We did not place Help or Contact Us links on the Webpage and thus wonder how many information needs went unmet because of that omission. Although our focus was on technology and information access; we acknowledge that basic human-to-human interaction is helpful.

g. Future iterations should identify and use a platform that incorporates technologies that allow push notifications or other automated dissemination of new search results.

h. We might have considered identifying key nursing journals to include on the Webpage.

i. We were heavily dependent on PubMed (Medline) because of its accessibility and familiarity but are aware it was not all inclusive.

Although we successfully formatted a Webpage for easy access to resources to guide EBP, we identified the need to increase the competency of our teams to evaluate and summarize the resources in order to make decisions based on an entire body of available evidence, rather than to rely on a single article or study. We also identified examples of decisions made without an evidence search. Some of the variabilities may be explained by chaos related to a worldwide pandemic but the variability highlighted the need to expand the culture of EBP at our institution. In early

2022, more than 20 health system nurse leaders completed a 40-hour EBP Immersion Workshop.[24] The workshop experience included practice with literature searches and tools to rapidly appraise and summarize relevant literature, as well as tools to synthesize the literature in such a way that recommendations may be visualized. Nurse leaders who attended the workshop are currently working with their individual teams to expand EBP competency and capacity.

We acknowledge the resources afforded to an academic medical center may not be available in other settings. Infectious microorganisms do not care if you have a library or library access. The need for efficient access to credible and translatable information is necessary for all health care workers, their families, and the public at large. Organizations without their own library can still replicate our actions with a small, dedicated team (formal or informal) of evidence-based champions or knowledge brokers.[25] Champions can perform an environmental scan on free or low-cost Web-based tools and seek approval within their organization. Although many organizations are familiar with intranets, they consider experimenting with social media platforms such as blogs[26] or wikis.[27] Information and guidance during infectious disease outbreaks are in a state of constant flux. The COVID-19 pandemic demonstrated that future pandemics would require health care personnel to participate in a living evidence ecosystem supported by integrated Internet and communication technologies that provide the right information at the right time to the right people.

SUMMARY

The speed of research and publishing brought many challenges to evidence-based practice and nursing care but none more paramount than the questions regarding the utility and futility of the traditional evidence-based paradigm during the pandemic. Information overload in health care is not a novel concept. However, the COVID-19 pandemic provides health care practitioners and information professionals an opportunity to revisit existing information management policies, strategies, architecture, and technologies to reduce the noise and deliver pertinent information in a systematic way that is effective, actionable, and tailored to its recipient. As we begin to prepare for the next pandemic, it will be crucial that we increase our competencies in accessing, rapidly appraising, and summarizing the evidence to make evidence-based decisions. Clinical nurses and nurse leaders must also start incorporating models and principles from the Information Sciences, Health Informatics, Communication Sciences, Health/Science Communication, and Information Ecology to effectively address the information needs of the health care workforce while staying empathetic to the demands of their workload and well-being.

Our project was a team-based initiative to reduce information seeking barriers by connecting nurses to strategically identified topics that were specifically related to the nursing context. By reducing obstacles such as time, resource awareness, searching skills, and other logistics we can instill confidence and comfort in knowing the workforce is applying the best possible care through informed decision-making and clinical decision support.[4,28,29] The *Nursing EBP for COVID-19* Webpage is a centrally located, well promoted, Web-based information resource that is user-friendly, independent of operating systems, and compatible with mobile or desktop devices. The development and constant revisioning of aggregated and vetted information from professional societies and associations and state and federal health authorities still left many information gaps for nurses and other health care practitioners. It was important to acknowledge the value of contextual primary research literature and identify methods to efficiently access it. Creating and saving search strings on the PubMed platform allows all health care organizations the ability to find primary literature within the Medline database. Furthermore, this approach connected users to thousands of *freely available full-text articles* related to COVID-19 in PubMed and PubMed Central that served as a viable supplement to the aggregated information from the State Department of Health, Centers for Disease Control and Prevention, and the World Health Organization.

Health care environments are dynamic and constantly changing, facts that are magnified when stressed by a global pandemic. As the largest segment of the health care workforce, the information needs of nurses must be supported so that nurses can consistently provide evidence-based care for their patients and maintain their own well-being.

CLINICS CARE POINTS

- Nurses are hungry for information needed to take care of their patients and themselves.
- The COVID-19 pandemic accelerated the need for evidence-based information, but information consumers must be competent to appraise and summarize the information.
- Evidence-based resources can be made available to health care workers without access to formal libraries.

DISCLOSURE

The authors have nothing to disclose.

ACKNOWLEDGMENTS

We would like to acknowledge the Health Sciences Informationists at the Eskind Biomedical Library, Camille Ivey; Heather Laferriere; and Rachel Walden, for their hard work and diligence with the search strings and their continued efforts with supporting the evidence-based practice culture of the Vanderbilt University Medical Center, United States.

REFERENCES

1. Chung BP, Wong TK, Suen ES, et al. SARS: caring for patients in Hong Kong. J Clin Nurs 2005;14(4):510–7.
2. Gebreselassie AF, Bekele A, Tatere HY, et al. Assessing the knowledge, attitude and perception on workplace readiness regarding COVID-19 among health care providers in Ethiopia-An internet-based survey. PLoS One 2021;16(3):e0247848.
3. González-Gil MT, González-Blázquez C, Parro-Moreno AI, et al. Nurses' perceptions and demands regarding COVID-19 care delivery in critical care units and hospital emergency services. Intensive Crit Care Nurs 2021;62:102966.
4. Lam SKK, Kwong EWY, Hung MSY, et al. Nurses' preparedness for infectious disease outbreaks: A literature review and narrative synthesis of qualitative evidence. J Clin Nurs 2018;27(7–8):e1244–55.
5. Norful AA, Rosenfeld A, Schroeder K, et al. Primary drivers and psychological manifestations of stress in frontline healthcare workforce during the initial COVID-19 outbreak in the United States. Gen Hosp Psychiatry 2021;69:20–6.

6. Shih FJ, Gau ML, Kao CC, et al. Dying and caring on the edge: Taiwan's surviving nurses' reflections on taking care of patients with severe acute respiratory syndrome. Appl Nurs Res 2007;20(4):171–80.

7. Kim Y. Nurses' experiences of care for patients with Middle East respiratory syndrome-coronavirus in South Korea. Am J Infect Control 2018;46(7):781–7.

8. El-Monshed AH, Amr M, Ali AS, et al. Nurses' knowledge, concerns, perceived impact and preparedness toward COVID-19 pandemic: A cross-sectional survey. Int J Nurs Pract 2021;27(6):e13017.

9. Prescott K, Baxter E, Lynch C, et al. COVID-19: how prepared are front-line healthcare workers in England? J Hosp Infect 2020;105(2):142–5.

10. Zhang M, Zhou M, Tang F, et al. Knowledge, attitude, and practice regarding COVID-19 among healthcare workers in Henan, China. J Hosp Infect 2020; 105(2):183–7.

11. Olum R, Chekwech G, Wekha G, et al. Coronavirus Disease-2019: Knowledge, Attitude, and Practices of Health Care Workers at Makerere University Teaching Hospitals, Uganda. Front Public Health 2020;8:181.

12. Sirois FM, Owens J. Factors Associated With Psychological Distress in Health-Care Workers During an Infectious Disease Outbreak: A Rapid Systematic Review of the Evidence. Front Psychiatry 2020;11:589545.

13. Hamric AB. Dealing with the knowledge explosion. Clin Nurse Specialist: J Adv Nurs Pract 2002;16(2):68–9.

14. MacGuire JM. Putting nursing research findings into practice: research utilization as an aspect of the management of change. J Adv Nurs 2006;53(1):65–71. Wiley-Blackwell.

15. Valika TS, Maurrasse SE, Reichert L. A Second Pandemic? Perspective on Information Overload in the COVID-19 Era. Otolaryngol - Head Neck Surg 2020; 163(5):931–3.

16. Casigliani V, De Nard F, De Vita E, et al. Too much information, too little evidence: is waste in research fuelling the covid-19 infodemic? BMJ (Clinical research ed) 2020;370:m2672.

17. Else H. How a torrent of COVID science changed research publishing - in seven charts. Nature 2020;553:7839.

18. Greenhalgh T. Will COVID-19 be evidence-based medicine's nemesis? PLoS Med 2020;6:e1003266.

19. Ioannidis JPA. Coronavirus disease 2019: The harms of exaggerated information and non-evidence-based measures. Eur J Clin Invest 2020;4:e13222.

20. Krouse HJ. Whatever Happened to Evidence-Based Practice During COVID-19? Otolaryngol Head Neck Surg 2020;163(2):318–9.

21. Makic MBF. Providing Evidence-Based Practice During the COVID-19 Pandemic. Crit Care Nurse 2020;40(5):72–4.

22. Watson R, McCrae N. Will evidence-based medicine be another casualty of COVID-19? J Adv Nurs 2020;12:3228–30.

23. Melnyk BM, Fineout-Overholt E, Gallagher-Ford L, et al. The state of evidence-based practice in US nurses: critical implications for nurse leaders and educators. J Nurs Adm 2012;42(9):410–7.

24. Helene Fuld Health Trust National Institute for Evidence-Based Practice in Nursing and Healthcare. Available at: https://fuld.nursing.osu.edu/. Accessed June 30, 2022.

25. Catallo C. Should Nurses Be Knowledge Brokers? Competencies and Organizational Resources to Support the Role. Nurs Leadersh (Tor Ont) 2015;28(1):24–37.

26. Blog. Cambridge Academic Content Dictionary. 2022. Cambridge: Cambridge University Press. Available at: https://dictionary.cambridge.org/us/dictionary/english/blog. Accessed November 22, 2022.
27. Wiki. Cambridge Academic Content Dictionary. 2022. Cambridge: Cambridge University Press. Available at: https://dictionary.cambridge.org/us/dictionary/english/wiki. Accessed November 22, 2022.
28. Brown RJL, Michalowski M. Nurses' Utilization of Information Resources for Patient Care Tasks: A Survey of Critical Care Nurses in an Urban Hospital Setting. Comput Inform Nurs 2022. https://doi.org/10.1097/cin.0000000000000908.
29. O'Boyle C, Robertson C, Secor-Turner M. Nurses' beliefs about public health emergencies: fear of abandonment. Am J Infect Control 2006;34(6):351–7.

Practical Implications of Online Learning with Nurses During Coronavirus Disease 2019

Collette Christoffers, MSN, RN, CNE*, Sara Bano, PhD,
Melissa Gorz, MEd

KEYWORDS

- Online • Nursing education • COVID-19 • RN-to-BSN • Self-care

KEY POINTS

- Although stressful and life changing, nursing faculty considered the COVID-19 pandemic a learning opportunity, not only for faculty but also for students.
- Recognizing and understanding emotional stress in online nursing students is an important factor in student success.
- Self-care should be prioritized to aid in work-life balance for faculty and students in online nursing programs.
- Professional development and institutional support can positively impact nursing faculty job satisfaction and student success in online nursing programs.

The coronavirus disease 2019 (COVID-19) pandemic severely tested health systems, hospital staff, and resources across the United States. As the largest health care profession, nurses have been challenged by surges in number of patients and shortages of patient care resources in addition to ethical and moral quandaries.[1] According to the American Nurses Foundation[2] COVID-19 Impact Assessment Survey (2022) 60% of acute care nurses reported feeling burned out, 75% reported feeling stressed, and 52% had considered or intended to leave the nursing profession. Although stress in the occupation of nursing has been well documented in past decades,[3,4] the COVID-19 pandemic brought concerns of physical and mental health to the forefront as nurses reported experiencing "burnout, exhaustion, and moral injury."[1] The emotional strain and stress of the COVID-19 pandemic was felt not only by nurses but also by their families; they had to navigate issues such as lack of childcare and school closures due to quarantine restrictions leading to conflicts in family responsibilities, professional obligations, and potential financial strain.[1]

School of Education, North Dakota State University, FLC 210, NDSU Dep. 2625, PO Box 6050, Fargo, ND 58108-6050, USA
* Corresponding author.
E-mail address: c.christoffers@ndsu.edu

Nurs Clin N Am 58 (2023) 107–119
https://doi.org/10.1016/j.cnur.2022.10.007
0029-6465/23/© 2022 Elsevier Inc. All rights reserved.

Furthermore, the impact of the COVID-19 pandemic extended into nursing education programs due to mandatory lockdowns implemented in March 2020. Much of the current literature about nursing education and the COVID-19 pandemic discusses the disruption of in-person classroom instruction and the impact for faculty and students moving abruptly to the online environment.[5–7] There is little to no empirical research available about how existing online nursing education programs were impacted by the pandemic. This study explores how faculty's perspectives, behaviors, and teaching practices changed in fully online nursing programs during the global COVID-19 pandemic.

LITERATURE REVIEW

Teaching nursing online is not a new development because nursing programs have leveraged current and emerging technologies to plan, deliver, and evaluate nursing education. Online distance education grew in the 1990s and proliferated in the early 2000s with advancement of the Internet. Registered Nurse to Baccalaureate (RN-to-BSN or Bachelor of Science in Nursing) program provides a bridge for diploma, and Associate Degree prepared nurses who wish to develop stronger clinical reasoning and analytical skills to advance their careers.[8] In 2019 the American Association of Colleges of Nursing (AACN)[8] reported that more than 78% of the RN-to-BSN programs across the United States were offered at least partially online. The offerings of RN-to-BSN completion programs are in response to disciplinary calls for a more highly educated workforce driven by the complex and changing health care environment.[9] Offering RN-to-BSN programs online enhances access for nurses to enroll in these programs.[8]

COVID-19 and Online Education

When the COVID-19 pandemic started, teaching online became a necessity around the world and many programs quickly transitioned to online learning to help control the spread of the virus.[5,7,10,11] Nursing programs that were already engaged with online learning also faced new challenges due to the pandemic.[10]

According to Lou and colleagues[12] in online nursing education, especially the RN-to-BSN program, additional challenges exist. A noted challenge is supporting working students' needs as they balance their professional, educational, and personal circumstances.[7] Students in online RN-to-BSN programs are often working in the industry as registered nurses. Owing to the COVID-19 pandemic, workloads for already busy nurses increased.[12] Shigemura and colleagues[13] predicted that health care workers would be required to work under harsher conditions such as longer working hours and unscheduled shifts because staff shortages would occur as co-workers became sick during the pandemic. This prediction became reality as the pandemic raged. Nurses found themselves working, often mandated, more days and longer shifts.[5]

In addition, working students also had to manage their coursework and family responsibilities. Online learning in a busy household can present challenges. In the study by Bdair[11], one participant noted being distracted by kids and other house obligations while studying at home. Some students reported increased stress caused by a combination of their coursework and family responsibilities.[14] Working students experienced increased worry about their family's health[12]; they expressed anxiety and fear related to the pandemic and the uncertainty of future events.[15] This situation further increased faculty workloads because they had to not only teach but also comfort students and provide them emotional support during the pandemic.[6]

Flexibility and Online Education

Online education brings many advantages such as convenience, flexibility, and speed for program completion.[10,16–18] However, online education also brings a wide range of challenges, including a considerable time commitment, difficulty engaging with students, difficulty with technology, lack of institutional support, and managing student expectations.[6,10,11,16,17,19]

Flexibility is seen as both an advantage and a disadvantage of online education. Bdair[11] found that students and faculty enjoyed the flexibility of online education and liked being able to participate in online learning at convenient times. In the study by Wingo and colleagues,[18] flexibility is noted as a distinct advantage to online nursing education, stating that busy faculty enjoyed online teaching because it let them participate in life activities and decide where and when to teach. In addition, flexibility comes from faculty being able to engage in their work at any time of the day or night. Some nursing faculty also reported that teaching online allowed them to continue working in the industry, and it also allowed them to travel to conferences while continuing their teaching.[17] For students, the flexibility afforded by online courses allows them to log in at their own convenience and work at their own pace.[10]

This flexibility also poses some problems for both faculty and students. Faculty sometimes feel they need to be always available because students may be working on course activities at all hours and on all days.[17] Students may become frustrated when faculty are not available to answer questions immediately.[20] Likewise, unreasonable expectations could be placed on the instructors by students and themselves.[18] There is also evidence that the flexibility offered by learning at home can actually decrease students' success and satisfaction. This decrease can occur due to lack of self-motivation and distractions at home, including the Internet, e-mail, and other daily tasks.[21] According to Bdair[11] students attending virtual classes from home sometimes lack motivation and are distracted by being in the home environment instead of a classroom.

Time Commitment in Online Education

There is a significant time commitment to developing and delivering online courses. In a study by Nabolsi and colleagues[6] participants expressed that the time faculty spent teaching online was much higher than the time they spent teaching face-to-face. While teaching online, faculty often have to respond multiple times to students' e-mails back and forth, which is generally more time consuming than face-to-face teaching.[17] Similarly, Puksa and Jansen[16] also argued in their study that a larger time commitment is needed for faculty teaching online courses, because participants in their study indicated that they felt like they never stopped and were constantly checking online posts. Furthermore, faculty mentioned that administration does not consider the workload expected of them and the additional time it takes to develop and deliver online courses.[10,16–18]

Overall, there are advantages and disadvantages of online teaching for faculty and students that can impact teaching and learning processes positively and negatively. As mentioned earlier, with the COVID-19 pandemic these challenges were exacerbated. In our study we tried to understand how nursing faculty navigated these challenges in an online nursing program and how they were able to support their students during the COVID-19 global pandemic.

RESEARCH QUESTIONS

1. How did nursing faculty navigate the impact of COVID-19 while teaching in the fully online environment?

2. How did nursing faculty support themselves and students (especially working in industry) as they adapted to the challenges brought by COVID-19?

RESEARCH DESIGN

For this study, a qualitative research design was used to help understand how nursing faculty teaching practices were impacted by COVID-19 in a fully online nursing program. Among the variety of the qualitative approaches, we chose Grounded Theory to guide data collection and data analysis processes. We used Grounded Theory because it is considered suitable for better understanding of a phenomenon.[22,23] Chun Tie and colleagues[24] argued that Grounded Theory methodology is appropriate to better understand a phenomenon and to construct an explanatory theory or concept to explain the process in a certain area of inquiry.

Context

We studied the experiences of faculty from a fully online RN-to-BSN nursing program at a 4-year institution in the upper-Midwest United States. The Upper Midwestern Institution (pseudonym) was established in 1889 and offers programs to prepare students for careers in business, health and physical fitness, psychology, science, mathematics, and nursing. The institution offers undergraduate and graduate degrees in aforementioned fields. In fall 2021, a total of 1200 students were enrolled with approximately 40% students participating in person and 60% in online education.

Participants

After institutional review board (IRB) approval of the study, we interviewed 7 nursing faculty members using purposeful sampling. All faculty members were female and taught in a fully online nursing program for registered nurses who have completed an associate degree and desire to continue their education to complete a bachelor's degree (RN-to-BSN program). According to Chun Tie and colleagues[24] purposeful sampling provides the initial data that researchers can use for analysis based on the Grounded Theory approach. The eligibility criteria included nursing faculty members who taught strictly in the online environment before, during, and after the COVID-19 pandemic in a fully online nursing program. See **Table 1** for participant demographic data.

Data Collection

We used semistructured informal interviews for data collection.[25] The interview protocol was developed to explore the online nursing faculty's teaching experiences in a

Table 1					
Participant demographics					
Alias	Years as RN	Years as Educator	Years as Online Educator	Full-Time Role	Part-Time Role
Ann	27	8	8	Associate professor	Faith community nurse
Barb	22	16	2	Nurse manager	Adjunct instructor
Connie	37	11	4	Associate professor	Staff educator in industry
Deb	18	4	4	Associate professor	Staff nurse in industry
Evie	24	12	4	Associate professor	Staff nurse in industry
Flora	26	2	2	Nurse manager	Adjunct instructor
Gabby	25	8	2	Associate professor	Clinic nurse practitioner

fully online nursing program during the COVID-19 pandemic. A pilot interview was conducted by 2 researchers to further refine the interview questions. The interview questions consisted of 9 open-ended questions with multiple follow-up questions (Appendix 1A for the research interview protocol). All interviews were conducted online using the Zoom platform in April 2022, and each interview lasted between 25 and 40 minutes.

Data Analysis

After the interviews were completed via Zoom, all files were saved in a password-secured shared Google Drive. The video interviews were transcribed. The transcripts were cleaned to remove extraneous filler words and identifiable data. All participants were assigned an alias to maintain confidentiality. The Grounded Theory approach was used for data analysis. Per Hutchinson[26] open coding consists of looking at each sentence and creating as many codes as possible to "ensure full theoretical coverage." Each researcher read and reread the transcripts and began their individual coding process. During this process, the researchers followed Hutchinson's[26] description of the constant comparative method, where analysts distinguish similarities and differences within the data. The researchers compared emerging codes, categories, and themes across all transcripts and established concepts in the literature. Finally, the researchers convened and examined the themes collectively.

Validity and Reliability

Several actions were taken to minimize the risk of researcher bias. For example, the research protocol was reviewed by all 3 researchers. IRB review and approval of the research protocol was obtained before the study. The researchers conducted a practice interview among the researchers to test the protocol and to allow for revisions of the protocol. Measures to increase the validity of the interview process included the researcher asking clarifying questions of the interviewees and reiterating statements for researcher understanding.

To ensure reliability, researcher triangulation was used for the data analysis process. Researchers cleaned the transcripts and listened to the interviews to ensure transcription accuracy. For the first round of data analysis, the transcripts were read by all researchers separately then reviewed for initial emerging themes. Researchers developed their separate codes and completed their data analysis process separately. During the second round of data analysis all researchers reviewed all the codes, categories, and themes to ensure consistency and to check biases in coding and the overall data analysis process.

FINDINGS

In this section we present our key findings from our study. Our main research questions were (1) how did nursing faculty teaching in the fully online environment navigate the impact of COVID-19 on their teaching practices and (2) how did they support themselves and their students during the pandemic? The following themes emerged from the data analysis process: perseverance and growth, humanizing teaching and learning practices, and resources for faculty success and development.

Perseverance and Growth

Many faculty members considered the COVID-19 pandemic a catalyst for change. The global pandemic pushed faculty to not only persevere in difficult circumstances but also transform their teaching practices. Faculty considered it an opportunity for personal and professional growth. Barb shared:

I think that [COVID-19 caused] a lot of growth …, you know, talk about doing impossible things. I see the good stuff that came out of that for a lot of people that I work with and maybe myself too, that there's things that probably [we] needed to work on anyway, and it just pushed it forward…I thought of World War II people, like my grandpa was World War II…and I thought of how long that lasted. There's been…disasters, and they've come out of it, and look at the great people…I mean they're known for that as a trait. That's an opportunity we have too (oral communication, April 2022).

The faculty members considered the COVID-19 pandemic a learning and growth opportunity not only for faculty but also for students; they believed that the pandemic pushed faculty to further improve their teaching practices. Deb shared:

I think the online courses were not disrupted as much as the in-person courses. We still got through our content. We maybe had to change it, but I think that content that was included or changed actually helped our students more than the content we were going to provide in the first place. They (students) were actually able to see boots on the ground, in real time, make those connections regarding the concepts. Obviously, nobody would want COVID-19 to happen, but I think in the aftermath we've learned a lot, and we have strength in the online programs (oral communication, April 2022).

The faculty members in our study considered the COVID-19 pandemic not only challenging but also an opportunity for growth for themselves and for their students. The faculty members also felt through perseverance they were able to improve their teaching practices and were able to support their students to achieve their academic goals in the challenging times of global pandemic.

Humanizing Teaching Practices

The faculty members in the online nursing program focused on humanizing the online learning experiences; they mentioned they were able to recognize and understand the emotional stress their students were going through due to the pandemic. The faculty members provided a variety of accommodations such as extension of deadlines, offering incompletes, and adjusting course content based on student needs. For instance, Connie explained:

with COVID-19 it was definitely a challenge with people getting assignments in, meeting timelines, meeting everything that was going…my goodness, because many of our students are rural students who were called into duty to work more hours because of COVID-19, take care of family because of COVID-19, ended up with COVID-19…we extended deadlines as much as we could. We changed activities…updated discussion questions to encourage them to talk about what they had been doing…so they could network in sharing with [nurses] in other areas (oral communication, April 2022).

Deb also shared similar experience:

I think it was a very emotional time…everyone was on high alert. Students reaching out…they were employed full time and saying 'I can't do all this. My kids are home now. I am working. I don't know the next time I'm going to be home…I'm trying to do my coursework.' I remember taking that feedback to our division of nursing, and we talked about it, and we said we need to give grace right now…we acknowledged that emotional piece because we were also suffering from [additional stress] and knowing that our students are trying to be everything to everyone at that moment (oral communication, April 2022).

The faculty members not only recognized and empathized with their students' challenges during the COVID-19 pandemic. Although it was an existing online program, the faculty members changed their approaches regarding course requirements and expectations to address the challenges of the pandemic to support their students.

Personal Strategies

Along with institutional support, the faculty members also mentioned personal strategies and resources that helped them navigate challenges of the COVID-19 pandemic in the online nursing program. These strategies included establishing professional boundaries and engaging in self-care.

Establishing professional boundaries: Being strictly in an online environment can make it difficult to maintain professional boundaries because students can reach out to faculty after regular business hours. All faculty members mentioned facing several challenges in maintaining professional boundaries especially at the start of the COVID-19 pandemic. Gabby shared her experience:

When you teach face to face, students ask the questions, but when you teach online, they ask the question whenever they're online for that class, and so I try to get back to them as soon as I can, which means that I'm checking my emails very often, much more often than I did before-getting back to them in the evenings, on the weekends, early hours, like whenever I see it, I try to respond to it (oral communication, April 2022).

All the faculty members in our study mentioned struggling with establishing boundaries, especially during the early phase of the pandemic. As Flora shared:

Initially, on my syllabus I had put my cell phone number down and then texting started to get abused...just a couple students, but it was enough to make me pull that back and really encourage them to use my email (oral communication, April 2022).

The faculty members learned to establish professional boundaries with time and experience; they considered learning to establish personal and professional boundaries a part of their learning process, which helped them take care of themselves and serve their students without feeling excessively overwhelmed during the pandemic.

Self-care: Self-care emerged as an important theme because almost all faculty members mentioned self-care as a key component of working through the impact of the COVID-19 pandemic. Similar to setting boundaries, it was a gradual learning process, because initially they found it difficult to practice self-care. Many of the faculty members made specific efforts to improve self-care practices. However, they believed they still needed to improve their self-care habits.

Deb shared her experience:

I feel like when [COVID-19] first started I was on my computer at all hours because I felt like I needed to be there for the students because they were struggling...knowing that they were the ones on the front lines, not me. I have incorporated a few self-care things into my courses. I do almost like a meditation reflection. It's guided imagery in my health promotions course that I do, and I walk through it (oral communication, April 2022).

Flora also shared similar experience:

There were very high stress levels....so self-care, honestly, during the COVID-19 pandemic for me was an afterthought. I've explored things like yoga, meditation, and different apps. The ANA did a pretty good job of putting self-care stuff out there (oral communication, April 2022).

Overall, faculty considered self-care and setting professional boundaries important in taking care of themselves and for supporting their students in the online learning environment during the global pandemic.

Institutional Resources

The faculty members mentioned different institutional resources that helped them in their online teaching practices. These resources included professional development opportunities, faculty collaboration, and mentorship.

Professional development: The topic of professional development was mentioned in 6 of the 7 online nursing faculty interviews as an appreciated resource provided by the institution. During the interviews, the faculty members frequently mentioned participating and benefiting from professional development activities provided by their institution during the COVID-19 pandemic. In particular, they mentioned a microcredentialing training by the Association of College and University Educators (ACUE). This training was a 25-week-long online microcredentialing course to teach faculty about best practices in the online education environment.

Evie (oral communication, April 2022) commented, "We got ACUE…I personally think I learned a lot and grew a lot and I think the online teaching environment improved because of that." Deb also shared that the ACUE training allowed her to "humanize" her online course because she learned to include a welcome video in her course. She mentioned, "From the [welcome] PowerPoint…I put my face out there every week so students can see [me]." Gabby (oral communication, April 2022) shared similar appreciation for this professional development opportunity, "going through the ACUE training to see evidence-based research about what students need in an online learning environment was very helpful." Overall, the faculty members in our study considered ACUE useful in navigating their teaching and learning during the COVID-19 pandemic because it provided them an opportunity to learn from experts in their field, communicate with their colleagues, and learn new strategies to use in their online courses.

In addition to the ACUE course, faculty also referred to other professional development opportunities such as offerings from the American Nurses Association, AACN, and NurseTim, which helped them improve their skills as educators in the online environment. Even though all faculty members interviewed had some experience teaching in the online environment, they felt the professional development resources and activities aided in their ability to enhance student engagement during the stressful time of the COVID-19 pandemic.

Faculty collaboration and mentorship: Faculty valued professional relationships and made an intentional effort to be collaborative and democratic with other nursing colleagues. Faculty discussed the importance of collaboration with other online nursing faculty and appreciated being assigned a specific mentor in their first 1 to 2 years of teaching online. Flora (oral communication, April 2022) elaborated the benefits of having a faculty mentor by saying "…having [a faculty mentor] assigned to me was incredibly helpful and not being thrown into doing something on my own right away-…everybody was very helpful." All faculty members emphasized that working collaboratively as a team not only enhanced their job satisfaction but also benefited their nursing students. Ann (oral communication, April 2022) shared, "Faculty met as a group to determine the best way to accommodate students and help alleviate some stress they were experiencing." Overall, the faculty members considered mentorship and faculty collaborations important for their success while teaching in the online environment during the pandemic.

To sum up, findings from our study suggest that the COVID-19 pandemic was challenging for the faculty members, but they still considered it an opportunity for personal and professional growth. The faculty used this disruption to reorient their teaching and humanize their teaching practices to support their students in the difficult times of a global pandemic. They also focused on incorporating self-care practices in their classes and in their lives. In addition, the faculty members embraced resources provided to them through professional development and mentorship and believed that institutional support was crucial for their personal and professional growth and persistence during the global pandemic.

DISCUSSION

Although our study focused on faculty who were teaching in the online environment before, during, and after the COVID-19 pandemic, our findings aligned with previous studies regarding increased challenges of teaching during the pandemic and supporting their online students. Similar to other studies, the faculty members in our study also acknowledged the increased workloads for already busy nursing students during the COVID-19 pandemic with longer working hours and unscheduled shifts.[5,12,13] Hrelic and Anderson[5] mentioned that faculty were considerate of the additional stress levels of their online students. In our study the faculty members shared the empathy they felt for their online students, which led them to collaborate with other nursing faculty to make necessary accommodations in the courses. The faculty members also shared experiences of supporting working students in balancing their professional, educational, and personal circumstances similarly noted by Oducado and Estoque.[7] Smith and colleagues[10] described establishing an online presence and providing encouragement for student engagement in the online learning environment.

In terms of change in teaching and learning practices, the nursing faculty interviewed focused on "humanizing" their teaching and learning practices; they mentioned some of their teaching strategies such as having a purposeful online presence, accommodating student needs, and personalizing discussion forums to encourage students to share their experiences. These strategies positively impacted student success and faculty satisfaction in the online environment. During the academic years 2020 and 2021, the overall program completion rate in the RN-to-BSN program was greater than 87%, which shows the success of the teaching strategies newly adopted by the faculty members. Also, these interventions by faculty are supported in the literature by Oducado and Estoque[7] as they argued that creating interventions to reduce stress among nursing students can help them cope with the academic challenges and work-related demands they face during the pandemic. Our findings support these claims, and we argue that humanizing online teaching and learning practices can positively contribute to student success.

Online nursing faculty interviewed in our study reiterated themes seen in the literature related to the flexibility and convenience of online education being both an advantage and disadvantage. Similarly to previous studies, our findings suggest that teaching online allowed faculty to continue working in the industry.[2,11,18] The faculty members also reported how this flexibility may also pose problems for both faculty and students because faculty feel they need to be always available because students are working on coursework at various times, and they do not want students to become frustrated at a slow response.[17,20] This tension led faculty to rethink work-life balance and focus on self-care. The COVID-19 pandemic changed faculty's attitudes toward self-care. Self-care emerged as an important theme from the faculty perspective and what they desired for their students as they taught in the online environment. The faculty members emphasized the importance of self-care and readily admitted they were "not good at self-care." Faculty interviewed in this study provided similar comments to the study by Gazza[17] in which participants mentioned "time is a blessing and a curse" and described the need to maintain work-life balance even when they wanted to be readily available to their online students. Faculty also were considerate of their students' life commitments and challenges during the COVID-19 pandemic, so they tried to incorporate self-care components in their teaching practices. We argue that self-care and work-life balance are important to ensure faculty and student success in the online environment. We have provided the self-care activities the faculty members in our study mentioned (see Appendix 1B).

In addition to personal strategies, our study highlights the significance of institutional support for faculty and student success. Wingo and colleagues[18] discussed how professional training programs can be challenging for faculty due to schedules, different training needs, and enthusiasm for training programs. Of the 7 faculty members interviewed in our study 6 spoke of the motivation to engage in professional development training sessions and appreciated the opportunities for professional development provided by their institution. Smith and colleagues[10] highlighted faculty have specific needs when teaching online. Among those needs include resources and administrative support.[10] Although the timing of the ACUE microcredentialing training may have added workload, professional development was highly valued by the faculty members interviewed in our study. Ignatavicius and Chung[27] argued that nursing faculty who participate in professional development transfer their newly acquired skills into educational practice. The faculty members in our study also shared how the ACUE microcredentialing training improved their ability to "humanize" their online learning environment. The faculty members also deeply valued the support they received from their mentors and from other nursing faculty. We argue that institutional support is crucial for faculty and student success and that institutions should provide regular professional development and mentorship opportunities to their faculty members.

To conclude, we suggest the following model in **Fig. 1** based on our findings. The model illustrates the conditions and interventions that contribute to working nursing students' success and nursing faculty satisfaction in online educational programs. In our study findings, faculty related to the student experience and used strategies to ensure a purposeful online presence. Faculty also collaborated with colleagues to accommodate student needs and allow for student sharing of experiences in the online environment. One final piece faculty described in our study was the concept of self-care. Self-care was described as a necessary component of faculty job satisfaction and student success.

RECOMMENDATIONS

This study illuminated several recommendations that faculty should consider as they teach nursing in the online environment. One set of recommendations revolves around

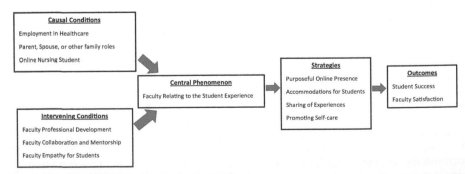

Fig. 1. Faculty relating to the student experience.

teaching methods and caring for students. Faculty should consider being flexible when teaching working nurses; they should also provide feedback, communicate openly, provide additional instructions to students, and embrace the technology that is available to them. In addition, it is important for faculty to model good self-care practices and encourage self-care in students. Faculty can also send positive messages to students, acknowledge student emotions, and give more grace to their working students.

Another set of recommendations is related to faculty support. When given the opportunity, faculty should participate in professional development being offered. In addition, they can collaborate with other faculty to ensure processes align between faculty. Furthermore, institutional investment into faculty should be encouraged and mentoring of new or junior faculty should be embraced.

A final set of recommendations concerns self-care practices. Throughout this study, faculty have illustrated the importance of participating in self-care activities, especially during stressful times such as the COVID-19 pandemic. Many faculty indicated they did not engage in as much self-care as they should. Suggestions for self-care include things like disconnecting from being online, interacting with others, embracing mindfulness, meditating, exercising, and having a personal mantra. These recommendations offer faculty a chance to enhance their teaching in online environments while also caring for themselves and students. See Appendix 1B for self-care suggestions as shared by participants in our study.

LIMITATIONS AND DELIMITATIONS

Our study has a small sample size, and all the participants were from the same institution and the same division, which limits generalizability to other fully online nursing programs. Another limitation of our study is that one of the researchers was a supervisor and part of the faculty group that was interviewed. This power differential may have impacted findings of our study. However, several measures were taken to minimize these risks of bias including piloting and revising the interview protocol and using researcher triangulation and theoretical sensitivity analysis as noted in the validity and reliability section.

CLINICS CARE POINTS

- Nurses need to reflect on the COVID-19 pandemic and share their stories to process their experience.
- Working nurses who engage in online education to advance their degree should look for self-care methods to aid in work-life balance and academic success.
- Support from others can positively impact nursing faculty job satisfaction and student success in online nursing programs.

DISCLOSURE

The authors have nothing to disclose.

SUPPLEMENTARY DATA

Supplementary data related to this article can be found online at https://doi.org/10.1016/j.cnur.2022.10.007.

REFERENCES

1. Chan GK, Bitton JR, Allgeyer RL, et al. The impact of COVID-19 on the nursing workforce: a national overview. Online J Issues Nurs 2021;26(2):1–17.
2. American Nurses Foundation. Pulse on the Nation's Nurses COVID-19 Survey Series: COVID-19 Impact Assessment Survey – The Second Year. 2022. Available at: https://www.nursingworld.org/practice-policy/work-environment/health-safety/disaster-preparedness/coronavirus/what-you-need-to-know/covid-19-impact-assessment-survey—the-second-year/. Accessed March 11, 2022.
3. Moustaka E, Constantinidis TC. Sources and effects of work-related stress in nursing. Health Sci J 2010;4(4):210–6.
4. Jennings BM. Work stress and burnout among nurses: role of the work environment and working conditions. In: Hughes RG, editor. Patient safety and quality: an evidence-based handbook for nurses. Agency for Healthcare Research and Quality; 2008. Available at: https://www.ncbi.nlm.nih.gov/books/NBK2668/. Chapter 26. Accessed March 17, 2022.
5. Hrelic DA, Anderson JG. Managing the unexpected: stressors and solutions for challenges experienced by RN-BSN students during an unprecedented global pandemic. J Prof Nurs 2022;40:48–56.
6. Nabolsi M, Abu-Moghli F, Khalaf I, et al. Nursing faculty experience with online distance education during COVID-19 crisis: a qualitative study. J Prof Nurs 2021;37(5):828–35.
7. Oducado RM, Estoque H. Online learning in nursing education during the COVID-19 pandemic: stress, satisfaction, and academic performance. J Nurs Pract 2021;4(2):143–53.
8. American Association of Colleges of Nurses. Degree completion programs for registered nurses: RN to master's degree and RN to baccalaureate programs. 2019. Available at: https://www.aacnnursing.org/Portals/42/News/Factsheets/Degree-Completion-Factsheet.pdf. Accessed April 8, 2022.
9. Institute of Medicine (US) Committee on the Robert Wood Johnson Foundation Initiative on the Future of Nursing, at the Institute of Medicine. The future of nursing: leading change, advancing health. Washington, DC: National Academies Press; 2011.
10. Smith Y, Chen Y-J, Warner-Stidham A. Understanding online teaching effectiveness: nursing student and faculty perspectives. J Prof Nurs 2021;37(5):785–94.
11. Bdair IA. Nursing students' and faculty members' perspectives about online learning during COVID-19 pandemic: a qualitative study. Teach Learn Nurs 2021;16(3):220–6.
12. Lou NM, Montreuil T, Feldman LS, et al. Nurses' and physicians' distress, burnout, and coping strategies during COVID-19: stress and impact on perceived performance and intentions to quit. J Contin Educ Health Prof 2022;42(1):e44–52.
13. Shigemura J, Ursano RJ, Kurosawa M, et al. Understanding the traumatic experiences of healthcare workers responding to the COVID-19 pandemic. Nurs Health Sci 2021;23(1):7–8.
14. Suliman WA, Abu-Moghli FA, Khalaf I, et al. Experiences of nursing students under the unprecedented abrupt online learning format forced by the national curfew due to COVID-19: a qualitative research study. Nurse Educ Today 2021;100:104829.
15. Bjester M, Cygan H, Morris Burnett G, et al. Faculty perspectives on transitioning public health nursing clinical to virtual in response to COVID-19. Public Health Nurs 2021;38(5):907–12.

16. Puksa MM, Janzen K. Faculty perceptions of teaching nursing content online in prelicensure baccalaureate nursing programs. J Nurs Educ 2020;59(12):683–91.
17. Gazza EA. The experience of teaching online in nursing education. J Nurs Educ 2017;56(6):343–9.
18. Wingo NP, Peters GB, Ivankova NV, et al. Benefits and challenges of teaching nursing online: exploring perspectives of different stakeholders. J Nurs Educ 2016;55(8):433–40.
19. Cole MT, Shelly DJ, Swartz LB. Online instruction, e-learning, and student satisfaction: a three-year study. Int Rev Res Open Online Education 2014;15(6): 111–31.
20. Culp-Roche A, Hardin-Fanning F, Tartavoille T, et al. Perception of online teacher self-efficacy: a multi-state study of nursing faculty pivoting courses during COVID 19. Nurse Educ Today 2021;106:105064.
21. Ladwig A, Berg-Poppe PJ, Ikiugu M, et al. Andragogy in graduate health programs during the COVID-19 pandemic. Distance Learn 2021;18(3):31–44. Available at: https://web-s-ebscohost-com.ezproxy.lib.ndsu.nodak.edu/ehost/pdfviewer/pdfviewer?vid=0&sid=169458af-8747-4c30-bf69-3441f8c36b66%40 redis. Accessed March 10, 2022.
22. Glaser BG. Theoretical sensitivity: advances in the methodology of grounded theory. Mill Valley, CA: Sociology Press; 1978.
23. Glaser BG. Basics of grounded theory analysis. Mill Valley, CA: Sociology Press; 1992.
24. Chun Tie Y, Birks M, Francis K. Grounded theory research: a design framework for novice researchers. SAGE Open Med 2019;7. 2050312118822927.
25. Creswell JW, Guetterman TC. Educational research: planning, conducting, and evaluating quantitative and qualitative research. 6th edition. New York, NY: Pearson; 2019.
26. Hutchinson SA. Education and grounded theory. J Thought 1986;21(3):50–68. https://www.jstor.org/stable/42589190. Accessed May 23, 2022.
27. Ignatavicius D, Chung CE. Professional development for nursing faculty: assessing transfer of learning into practice. Teach Learn Nurs 2016;11(4):138–42.

Moving?

Make sure your subscription moves with you!

To notify us of your new address, find your **Clinics Account Number** (located on your mailing label above your name), and contact customer service at:

Email: journalscustomerservice-usa@elsevier.com

800-654-2452 (subscribers in the U.S. & Canada)
314-447-8871 (subscribers outside of the U.S. & Canada)

Fax number: 314-447-8029

Elsevier Health Sciences Division
Subscription Customer Service
3251 Riverport Lane
Maryland Heights, MO 63043

*To ensure uninterrupted delivery of your subscription, please notify us at least 4 weeks in advance of move.

Printed and bound by CPI Group (UK) Ltd, Croydon, CR0 4YY

03/10/2024

01040469-0010